Baby Biorhythms and Breastfeeding

Maria Galles

ISBN 978-1-5059-0866-4

Cover Art includes Frosted Dark Green Pattern Background Image
Free Use, compliments of Eileen with EZTechTraining.com

This book is not intended as a substitute for the medical advice of a physician.
The reader should consult a physician particularly with respect to any symptoms,
signs of illness, or any unusual behavior that may require diagnosis or medical attention.

Although the author and publisher have made every effort to ensure that the
information in this book was correct at press time,
the author and publisher do not assume and hereby disclaim any liability
to any party for any loss, damage, or disruption caused by errors or omissions,
whether such errors or omissions result from negligence,
accident, or any other cause.

First printing March 2015
10 9 8 7 6 5 4 3 2 1

DEDICATION

I dedicate this book to:

my mom, Mary

my wonderful husband, Bob

and to my eight breastfed babies:
Laura, Veronica, Zachary, Nathan,
Daniel, Calvin, Teresa and Jacob

Thank you to
Bob, Deb, Julie, Diane, Susan, Laura, and Zach
for all their help in making this book possible

May God bless you, the reader,
in this awesome commitment to motherhood!

bi·o·rhythm
/ˈbīōˌriT͟Həm/

noun

noun: **biorhythm**; plural noun: **biorhythms**;
noun: **bio-rhythm**; plural noun: **bio-rhythms**

1. a recurring cycle in the physiology or
functioning of an organism, such as the
daily cycle of sleeping and waking.
   ○ a cyclic pattern of physical, emotional,
   or mental activity said to occur in the life
   of a person.

Define biorhythm - Google Search. (n.d.). Retrieved March 1, 2015,
from www.google.com/search?q=define+biorhythm

TABLE OF CONTENTS

Preface

Everyone should have a passion for something in life. One of my passions is the importance of breastfeeding. I am adamant about the benefits of breastfeeding: not just for baby, but for mom as well.

Baby Biorhythms and Breastfeeding is for women who are serious about breastfeeding. Moms who make the decision to breastfeed are often challenged to navigate in unclear and unchartered waters. In a society that continues to demand more of our time, moms question: "is there a way to find balance between breastfeeding and the rhythm of daily life?" The answer—"Yes, there is!"

To help make breastfeeding successful, this book shares the rewards of breastfeeding, how to prepare before baby arrives, and the benefits of establishing a daily routine for both baby and mom. It includes a reference guide of the feeding, sleeping, and weaning biorhythms of our own children from birth through age one and beyond.

In journaling the feeding routines and sleeping patterns of our babies over the past 10+ years, I have discovered definite rhythmic patterns of eating and sleeping. Learning about your baby's biorhythms and adjusting these biorhythms along with your own can help take the guesswork out of what your baby needs. In return, this knowledge and experience will hopefully help you become more confident and relaxed parents. I encourage you to clasp onto the buoy of *Baby Biorhythms and Breastfeeding*, and use it as a compass to guide you along this breastfeeding journey!

With our first daughter, my husband, Bob, and I didn't know a lot about breastfeeding or its commitment. Once our second daughter arrived, we realized the importance of forming a regular breastfeeding routine with our children. This routine of feedings, naptimes, and bedtime allowed us to know what our babies needed and when they needed it. Soon after, adjusting baby's natural biorhythms with our own adult biorhythms led to our babies sleeping through the night and more time together as a couple.

Bob and I also discovered that synchronizing our resting, sleeping, and eating patterns with our baby's patterns reduced our anxiety, increased our confidence, and led to greater harmony in our home. Being able to find a new normal and being flexible to our baby's biorhythms were keys to finding what works best in our family.

I wrote *Baby Biorhythms and Breastfeeding* during the spare moments and waiting times of life—naptimes, doctor's office visits, and carpool to name a few. This guide reflects my personal experience of eight normal, full term pregnancies. Please use *Baby Biorhythms and Breastfeeding* as a supplemental guide—seek professional advice with your ob/gyn, pediatrician, family doctor, and/or certified lactation consultant with any questions or concerns you have about breastfeeding to get personal advice based on your specific situation.

In Titus 2:4, the Greek word *philoteknos* appears in reference to mothers loving their children.[5] The meaning is expressed beautifully by GotQuestions Ministries in these words:

> *"This word represents a special kind of 'mother love.' The idea that flows out of this word is that of caring for our children, nurturing them, affectionately embracing them, meeting their needs, and tenderly befriending each one as a unique gift from the hand of God"*[8]

God bless you for the time, effort, commitment, and love you have for your child!

Maria R. Galles

Introduction: Why Breastfeed?

So you've make the big decision to breastfeed? If so, hats off to you! God has designed women to bear and nourish their children so you're making a great choice! Perhaps you're reading this book because you're not certain about whether or not you plan to breastfeed and would like to learn more. Excellent! I thank you for your consideration in the matter.

Here are some of the breastfeeding benefits for baby:
1. Your baby will have better antibodies and fewer illnesses from breast milk. Children who benefit from the antibodies in breast milk have been shown to exhibit lower respiratory infections and fewer occurrences of asthma, obesity, and type 2 diabetes. Breast milk has also been shown to lower the risk of SIDS or sudden infant death syndrome.[19]

2. Your baby is receiving the best nutrition from breast milk.[19]

3. Breast milk is gentler on baby's stomach than formula.

4. Your baby benefits immensely from the close bonding time with mom.[18]

Here are some benefits of breastfeeding for mom:
1. Breastfeeding can help mom's uterus to contract and shrink mom's tummy more quickly.

2. Mom will enjoy this quiet and close bonding time with baby. She can sit back, put her feet up and truly enjoy being in the presence of her child.

3. Mom will marvel and appreciate the creation of the female body and God who gifted her with the ability to provide a safe haven where her baby can live and grow.

4. Mom will marvel at the fact that God created her to provide nourishment for her baby.

5. Mom will save money by not having to buy expensive baby formula.

6. Mom will save money and time by not having to purchase baby bottles and wash them regularly.

7. Mom will not have to worry about having to bring and pack baby bottles and formula for outings.

8. Mom's overall health can be improved by breastfeeding. "Breastfeeding is linked to a lower risk of these health problems in women: Type 2 diabetes, breast cancer, ovarian cancer, and postpartum depression." [19]

9. Mom will be able to demonstrate *philoteknos* through breastfeeding. "Breastfeeding can feel great. Physical contact helps newborns feel more secure, warm, and comforted. Moms can also benefit from this closeness. Breastfeeding requires mom to take some quiet time to relax and bond with baby. This skin-to-skin contact can boost the mom's oxytocin levels. Oxytocin is the hormone that helps milk flow and calms mom." [19]

   Oxytocin is the "letdown" hormone. It produces relaxed and sleepy-calm feelings for mom in response to baby's sucking at the breast.[12] Prolactin is the hormone released during breastfeeding. It is responsible for milk production. Prolactin is sometimes called "the love hormone" and has been attributed to mothering behaviors. Like oxytocin, prolactin appears to produce a calming effect for mothers.[3]

Biorhythms: The Benefits of Balance and Daily Routine

As adult human beings, we are creatures of habit and routine. We sleep a certain number of hours per night. We eat a certain number of times per day and at certain regular intervals. For most of us, daytime is when we are most awake and effective. It is when we work and play. Nighttime is typically the time to rest and rejuvenate our bodies so we can begin again a new day of activity tomorrow.

God designed our bodies and their biorhythms. We know from experience that it's hard to do anything well if one is not listening to his/her biorhythmic needs for sleep and healthy sustenance. If such needs are important for adults, it is logical that a baby would benefit from following a biorhythmic routine as well.

As the managers of the home, it is important for parents to establish a routine format. A breastfeeding and sleeping routine allows mom and dad to know when their baby is hungry, when their baby is tired, and how to satisfy those needs in a manner that keeps baby satisfied and content. Recognizing the biorhythms of your baby and synchronizing these biorhythms with your own biorhythms as parents allows you to be a more confident parent that knows what baby's needs are and how to address them.

As a new mom, I didn't really have a clue about how to breastfeed a baby, how often babies need to breastfeed, how often a baby naps, or when a baby should nap. Ever since the birth of our second child, my husband and I began to take note of the importance of a regular breastfeeding, napping, and bedtime routine.

In our experience, it seemed that our first child cried more than her siblings. Maybe she was just crankier or more colicky than our other children. Looking back, my husband and I believe she may have picked up on our own insecurities and anxieties as new parents. This probably made her more edgy. Thinking she must be hungry, I breastfed her—or tried to—whenever she cried. We really didn't know when she was tired, hungry, or when she needed a diaper change—except for obvious reasons.

She had no normal bedtime, naptime, or breastfeeding routine. After about three months of our baby waking up and crying several times throughout the night, my husband and I were exhausted. We were tired, cranky, and frustrated parents. Breastfeeding was not appearing to be as great as all the books and advocates claimed. We tried to soothe her with an audiocassette tape of a heartbeat set to lullaby songs...that didn't work. We paced with her for hours...that didn't work either. We rocked with her on the rocking chair until she finally fell asleep—only to startle herself back awake as we tried to lay her down in her crib. Thus began the wailing again. Finally we were so fried, tired, and frazzled that we did the unthinkable—we let our baby cry it out until she settled herself down and fell asleep. This is the point where we reached our epiphany as parents and the first sleeping and feeding routines began.

Once, while on a moms' retreat, a religious sister told us story. It was about a mother and her young son traveling by airplane. During the flight, there was a failure of cabin air pressure. An oxygen mask deployed over her seat, but not over the seat of her son. The mother's first instinct was to grab her own oxygen mask and put it over her son's face to keep her child conscious. Pondering just a few seconds more, she took the mask and put it over her own face first. Why did she decide to do this? The mother knew that if she went unconscious first she would not be able to help her own child. Her child was too young to understand what was best for him to do. By the mother breathing the air first and retaining consciousness, she was able to help her child by comforting him and attending to his needs by sharing her oxygen mask with him.

I never really thought much about this story again until I began to write this book. A good mother doesn't have to give all or nothing to her child. Sometimes to be a good mother, we have to make sure our needs our being taken care of first so we are happy and healthy enough to take care of the needs of our child. Often, a breastfeeding and sleeping routine can foster harmony and balance between both baby's and mom's biorhythms.

Getting Ready: Am I Committed?

The amount of time mothers have to nurture and nourish their children by breastfeeding goes so quickly. The female body is amazing in its divine design to protect and nourish its young. New mothers may be concerned that breastfeeding will change their life and the way they do things. It most certainly will—and for the better. Like anything worthy of doing or achieving, breastfeeding takes time and commitment.

At times, I have felt limited in where I could go and what I could do before I had to be home in time for the next nursing. Now, I look back and cherish the bonding time I shared with my children through breastfeeding. I love the time I can excuse myself from busyness, company, and household tasks to sit, relax, and give nourishment and comfort to my baby.

I'm not going to lie to you—breastfeeding can be difficult. At the beginning you may experience breast engorgement (overfilling of the breasts with milk), the pain of uterine cramping, the discomfort of baby latching on to the breast, chapped nipples, and sleep deprivation. However, if you can persevere through the first 2 to 4 weeks as a beginning breastfeeding mother, I assure you that breastfeeding becomes so much easier and you'll be glad you stuck with it. In a society that endorses "it's all about me," not being inconvenienced and not offending anyone, I challenge you to swim against the current and do what is best for your baby—breastfeeding!

Many moms have good intentions of breastfeeding after their baby is born and plan on doing so for a while. Unfortunately, fear of the unknown, insecurity, and inexperience result in moms going to the bottle—for baby that is.

For example, a 2006 survey reported that 80% of women before delivery indicated that they intended to breastfeed. By the end of baby's first week after birth, 50% of the women had already given their baby infant formula. At nine months, only 35% of these women were breastfeeding to any extent.[2]

Another report from the Centers for Disease Control and Prevention showed that although more U.S. moms are breastfeeding their infants, few continue to do so for the recommended 12 months. From 2000–2008 fewer than half of the infants in the survey were still being breastfed at six months.[16]

"Many mothers who want to breastfeed are still not getting the support they need from hospitals, doctors, or employers. We must redouble our efforts to support mothers who want to breastfeed," said Dr. Tom Frieden, Director of the CDC.[15]

Dr. Claire McCarthy echoes the need for support for breastfeeding moms. A recent study in the journal *Pediatrics* in 2012 says only one third of moms who plan on exclusively breastfeeding for three months or more actually do so.[13]

After reviewing the statistics above, you may be asking yourself, "Why do moms quit breastfeeding?" According to Pediatrician Dr. Claire McCarthy, there are four common reasons why moms stop breastfeeding. These reasons include a rough start, worry that baby isn't getting enough milk, discomfort with nursing in public, and having to go back to work.[13] Let's look deeper into these four reasons why moms quit breastfeeding.

To reiterate what was mentioned at the beginning of this chapter, breastfeeding is definitely hard work at first. Breast engorgement, the pain of uterine cramping, the discomfort of baby latching on to the breast, chapped nipples, and sleep deprivation are definite challenges for new moms. However, if you persevere beyond those first 2 to 4 weeks as a beginning breastfeeding mother, I assure you that breastfeeding will become so much easier!

Another concern new moms have is "Is baby getting enough?" Dr. McCarthy is right on when she says, "We are a bottle culture. When we don't see how much our baby drinks, we get nervous." It is true that breastfed babies eat more often than formula fed babies since breast milk is easily digested and moves quickly through the digestive system. Because breast milk is more easily digested, breastfed babies get hungrier sooner than bottle-fed babies. Mom's worry that baby isn't getting enough due to getting hungry sooner often results in formula supplementation.

Dr. Claire McCarthy states, "If baby is eating at least every 3 hours or so, wetting at least 6 diapers in 24 hours, pooping regularly, and mom sees baby swallowing, baby is most likely getting enough." [13] Other hindrances that go along with mom's worry of baby getting enough are unsolicited negative comments from society. Comments such as "Are you *still* nursing?", "Maybe your milk isn't enough, why don't you add formula?", and "Your baby still seems hungry" are definitely not confidence boosters for new moms who want to breastfeed. Mom, do your best to blow off such negative comments made by know-it-alls.

A third reason why moms quit breastfeeding is the discomfort with nursing in public. Since we are a bottle culture, women often feel or are made to feel uncomfortable nursing their baby in public. Being able to master this hurdle of the mind with confidence can be a challenge. Some may view breastfeeding as offensive and unnecessary for moms to be whipping out their breasts in public to feed their babies. You can be more modest about breastfeeding by using a blanket or hooter hider (a cover that mom wears while nursing her baby that looks similar to a stylish apron that hangs around mom's neck) to cover up your unmentionables during a feeding.

Let's face it, moms are busy. We cannot be expected to never leave our homes just because our breastfeeding may offend someone. The faster you can get over your shyness to breastfeed within the family and public, the better. This may be difficult, but if I can do it, so can you!

A final common reason why moms quit breastfeeding is having to go back to work. Returning to work after the birth of a baby can be stressful. Finding the time and place to pump breast milk along with the storing and transporting of breast milk deter many moms from continuing breastfeeding upon their return to work.[13]

By and large, we know the tremendous benefits of breastfeeding. So what is the solution in creating a culture that promotes breastfeeding? It is **support** and **education**. Hospitals need to support, encourage, and educate breastfeeding moms as do ob/gyns, pediatricians, and family doctors. Better promotion of breastfeeding before baby is born is needed so that parents are prepared, and the decision to breastfeed has already been made before baby's birth. Breastfeeding moms need the support of their families, one another, and their community.

The AAP recommends exclusive breastfeeding for about six months, with continuation of breastfeeding for 1 year or longer as mutually desired by mother and infant.[4] This recommendation is concurred by the World Health Organization and The Institute of Medicine. This book is designed to walk mothers through a one-year commitment to breastfeeding. Maybe your commitment to breastfeeding is six months or maybe it is nine months. Whatever you decide, use this book as a guide. Always consult your baby's doctor or a lactation consultant with questions and concerns you have about breastfeeding and baby's nutritional needs.

So I ask you to decide: are you ready to commit to breastfeeding your baby? If you decide yes—that's awesome! I commend your resolve to provide your baby with the best nutrition possible—God's divine drink for babies!

Planning Ahead: What Do I Need to Make Breastfeeding Successful?

As a naïve first-time mother, I thought all I had to do in order to make breastfeeding a success was attend a class about it and give birth. Boy, was I mistaken! Don't get me wrong, the breastfeeding class was extremely helpful, but watching a movie about breastfeeding and practicing techniques with a doll are just not the same thing as breastfeeding a real baby.

Like any job, to do it well, one needs the proper tools, practice, repetition, and training. So what do you really need to make breastfeeding a success? Preparation and perseverance! If you have the knowledge and tools you need to make breastfeeding a success, it will be. Here are my top 15 ways to be prepared:

1. **Attend a breastfeeding class at your hospital a few months before your baby is due.** The lactation consultants are knowledgeable and enthused about breastfeeding and can answer all of your questions.

2. **Make or purchase a set of cheap and comfortable stretchy/elastic bracelets to go with several wardrobe outfits.** This bracelet will be necessary later to keep track of which breast you left off at the last nursing so you can resume the next feeding at that breast. Hair scrunchies may serve this purpose as well. Knowing and remembering with which breast you concluded the feeding is essential for good milk flow and breast comfort when beginning another feeding. This little bracelet is a lifesaver when you're tired and can't remember which breast you left off to start the next feeding!

3. **Buy at least four nursing bras and several sets of nursing bra pads a couple of months before baby is due.** To reduce cost and waste, I personally like the cotton washable nursing pads. There are disposable pads as well. Like regular bras, nursing bras come in all types of styles—wireless, underwire, sport, clip down, and wrap to name a few. Ask a girlfriend, sister, cousin, aunt, or mother that has breastfed to go shopping with you and help you choose a good and comfortable fit and style. Ask a maternity sales clerk to help you with recommendations and styles of nursing bras and try them on before purchasing.

   Once you get home, wash and wear these bras to get comfortable wearing them before baby is born. I recommend buying extra nursing bras and pads. Once your milk comes in after baby is born (usually about 3–5 days post-partum) your breasts will leak as your milk supply adjusts to baby's demands. Having extra nursing bras and nursing pads will come in handy due to their needed daily laundering. You may also want to consider a nursing night gown or nursing sleep top and some comfortable bedtime nursing bras. No one ever told me that I would pretty much need to wear a nursing bra of some sort 24 hours per day!

4. **Purchase or rent a breast pump from a local department store or your hospital lactation consultant.** I personally like the manual Avent breast pump. There are several on the market so do some research and ask a lot of questions—especially with your hospital's lactation consultant. Also, check with your insurance to see if buying or renting breast pumps is included or discounted with your medical coverage.

5. **Purchase a nursing pillow.** This is a U-shaped pillow that sits on mom's lap, goes around her waist, and helps support baby during breastfeeding. A popular brand is Boppy. You may want two—one for baby's bedroom and one for another common feeding area in the home. This way you won't have to constantly remember to carry the nursing pillow back and forth or up and down stairs when it is time for a feeding. There are also slip covers made for nursing pillows to protect the pillow and make laundering easier.

6. **Establish a nursing station.** Decide where you will regularly nurse your baby. My nursing station is a gliding rocker in baby's room. Other crucial tools at my nursing station are my nursing foot stool, a water bottle or cup for mom, and my nursing pillow. You may choose to set up a secondary nursing station somewhere else in your home as well, for ease and convenience. My secondary nursing station is my recliner in the living room.

7. **Purchase a nursing foot stool.** My nursing foot stool is in baby's room next to the gliding rocker. It provides good support and lifts my legs up so baby fits comfortably on the nursing pillow and is lifted high enough to reach the breast without my arms having to be flexed or strained to provide constant support during a feeding.

8. **Purchase extra maxi-pads.** While breastfeeding, your uterus will continue to cramp and cause the continuation of blood flow for about a month after delivery.

9. **Have comfortable cold compresses and lanolin for breastfeeding mothers on hand.** The compresses should be refrigerated and may be applied to your breasts to help relieve any engorgement those first few weeks postpartum. The lanolin will soothe chapped nipples from baby latching on.

10. **Ask your health care professional about pain medication you may take while breastfeeding.** Have that pain medication already on hand in your medicine cabinet at home to help manage uterine cramping pains.

11. **Have a water bottle or cup readily available for you at your home nursing station.** Lactating moms need more water to produce milk for baby. Drink water before you begin your nursing session. To help prepare, refill your water before you go to bed at night and again in the morning. This is something you can ask your husband to do or even assign another child in the home to do for you as part of their daily chores. If you have a secondary nursing station near the center of your home's activity—mine being the kitchen, have a full water bottle or cup on the kitchen counter that is always ready and waiting for you. Fill it in the morning and the afternoon so it is always there for you to drink.

12. **If you have a split level home with baby's room upstairs, consider having a portable crib on the main floor for napping and diaper changes.** This will avoid constant trips up and down the stairs for sleep-deprived moms those first couple of months.

13. **Have a watch or clock handy.** This is essential for helping you know when baby nurses and for how long.

14. **Keep a pen and paper handy to log the number of times per day your baby is nursing.** This will help you avoid having to rely on your memory to track the number of times your baby is nursing per day in your sleep-deprived state.

15. **Read this book in its entirety.**

16. **Re-read each chapter in advance of making it to baby's next monthly milestone.**

17. **Re-read each chapter again when you reach the applicable month.**

Beyond Spock: Changes in Education

Most people would agree that the childcare "bible" for parents in the 1950s–1970s was Dr. Benjamin Spock's *Baby and Child Care*. From the late 1980s through today, the childcare "bible" for parents shifted to the Murkoff, Mazel, Eisenberg, and Hathaway *What to Expect* series. The changes in education during the past 60 years have been phenomenal. Even in raising our own children over the last 15 years, there have been marked changes in what has been deemed "best" in infant and child care. It is no wonder that our parents think we are nuts when we do the things we do 'in the best interest' of our children and vice versa.

Dr. Spock advised our parents and grandparents that it was best to lay infants down to sleep on their stomachs, cover infants with a blanket in the crib, start baby on ground meats between 2–6 months of age and egg yolks between 5–6 months of age.[17] Today parents are advised lay infants down on their backs to sleep to prevent SIDS (Sudden Infant Death Syndrome), to use sleep sacks instead of blankets in the crib, and avoid bumper pads and toys in the crib.[14] As far as diet goes, since 2012 the AAP recommends exclusive breastfeeding of infants to 6 months of age.[4] The reasoning behind this is less allergies and easier digestion for infants. These are just a few examples of the changes in education for parents within the past generation or two, or even in the same generation.

With our family's children born before 2012, we followed the AAP's recommended beginning of rice cereal and baby food between the ages of 4–6 months. After 2012 we follow the new AAP guidelines with exclusive breastfeeding until 6 months. This book, *Baby Biorhythms and Breastfeeding*, reflects the updated and current AAP guidelines.

Infant and child care information and recommendations are always changing. Hopefully that is because we are smarter and have the best information available. Keep yourself educated of the changes in infant and child care to keep your baby safe, healthy, and happy.

Biorhythms: Observing Patterns and Transition Signs

The key to forming a happy and healthy biorhythm between you and your baby lies in observing the patterns and transition signs in baby's eating and sleeping habits. Establishing a biorhythmic routine will help create an environment of awareness, strengthen parental confidence, and take the guesswork out of what baby needs and when baby needs it.

No mother and child pair will have the exact same biorhythm or do things at the same time of day or chronological age as other mothers and their babies. Every child is a unique gift from God, and each family has its own circumstances and environment. However, meshing baby and mom's biorhythms together will help them live in better harmony. You're being called to embrace change, discover new norms, and embark on this exciting new adventure together!

Through journaling my children's patterns of eating and sleeping for the past 10 years, I have observed many consistencies. These biorhythmic patterns and transitions are detailed throughout the following chapters, and summarized in the appendix at the end of the book. Note that the patterns may vary for each child—this book is a general account of our children. Take note of the signs and adjust as needed for your own baby—seek baby's cues and use your own observations to confirm when your baby is "ready" to transition and take the next step.

God, grant me . . .

The **serenity** *to accept the things I cannot change,*

The **courage** *to change the things I can,*

and the **wisdom** *to know the difference.*

\- Reinhold Niebuhr

The First Month: Beginning Breastfeeding

Congratulations on the birth of your child! Well, you did it. You made it through labor and delivery and have a beautiful baby! Well done!

Remember to let those feelings of joy and elation shine through—even in the midst of changing lots of diapers and breastfeeding every 2–3 hours. Marvel at your precious child and the gift of motherhood. God designed the female body wonderfully to carry life in the womb and provide sustenance for this precious gift of life.

The first month post-partum is what really makes or breaks a breastfeeding mother. It **is** the most difficult month. This is why pre-planning before baby's arrival and an awareness of what to expect are essential. By reading this book, *Baby Biorhythms and Breastfeeding*, you will feel less baffled and less frustrated about breastfeeding and what to expect once baby is born.

While pregnant, your body has changed dramatically in preparation for motherhood. Your body will continue to change after birth. Within a few days post-partum, your milk will come in. While at the hospital, breastfeed baby within the first hour after baby is born. Feed baby frequently the first few days to establish your milk supply. Take advantage of your lactation consultant. Don't hesitate to call on your lactation consultant or attending breastfeeding nurse each time you feed your baby to confirm a proper "latch-on" (when baby's mouth attaches to the breast to nurse) or to ask any other questions. So maybe you feel a little strange asking a stranger to look at your breast and tell you if your baby is "latched-on" properly. This is perfectly normal. Up to this point in our lives, breasts have really only been viewed by society as sexual and not maternal. This is the point where you're experiencing a huge paradigm shift. Remember, God designed the female body to be amazing and the true purpose of the breast is for moms to provide sustenance for their child(ren). So take a deep breath and ask your lactation consultant lots of questions. Believe me, lactation consultants are thrilled with your questions and glad that moms like you want to do what is best for their babies by breastfeeding. Take advantage of your time in the hospital with the resources that are available. Go ahead and press that nurse call button.

When you're discharged from the hospital and want to continue to confirm proper breastfeeding, contact your lactation consultant. She will have support information, provide baby weigh-ins to check proper weight gain, and be able to provide information about joining a breastfeeding support group such as La Leche League or something similar in your area. La Leche League is an international nonprofit organization that distributes information on and promotes breastfeeding. "La Leche" means "milk" in Spanish. Check out the La Leche League website online at www.llli.org for more great information about breastfeeding or to find a local breastfeeding support group.

So baby has arrived and what should you do now? What should you expect? Know that the first two weeks post-partum can be the most difficult. Just remember to stick to your guns about your commitment to breastfeeding.

Before you begin this breastfeeding adventure, please consider these four questions:

1. What can mom expect?

2. What does baby need?

3. What does mom need?

4. What support can dad or the family provide?

What can mom expect?

Mom, first let's consider expectations for you. Your milk will generally come in around day three (give or take). In the meantime, baby is getting just what is needed from the colostrum you provide. Colostrum is the pre-milk substance—rich with protein and antibodies—that baby drinks from mom the first few days after birth until mom's milk is ready. It is very important to feed baby within the first hour of birth and to feed frequently those first few days to help establish an overall milk supply. Your baby will benefit from that close skin to skin contact with mom.

Watch for feeding cues of rooting— when baby moves the head back and forth and opens the mouth in search of mom's breast—so you can tell when your baby is hungry. While breastfeeding, try to observe how and when baby slows down or ceases feeding at one breast and is ready to start feeding at the other.

Those first few breastfeeding weeks are the most challenging. You will be ready to go through the roof at latch-on. Why? The reasons for discomfort are breast engorgement caused from increased milk supply, and chapped and sore nipples from repeated latch-on. There are things that can relieve the pains of breast engorgement and chapped nipples. Place soft ice packs in your bra to help relieve the swollenness of the breasts. Lanolin cream will help soothe and heal chapped nipples.

Try not to pump or express breast milk during those first 4 weeks post-partum. If you need to pump due to extreme engorgement, that is fine. Not expressing or pumping breast milk will allow your body to self-regulate its milk supply and not think it needs to overproduce. Ask your lactation consultant about other remedies to relieve engorgement and about creams that can be applied to chapped nipples.

In addition to sore breasts and nipples, be prepared to feel pain from uterine cramping while you're breastfeeding. Breastfeeding does cause the uterus to contract—which is good for you because you'll shed that extra baby weight sooner, but the resulting cramping will cause discomfort. In addition to physical discomfort, your post-partum hormones are running rampant resulting in a myriad of emotions. Pay attention to how you feel. Be proactive about your physical and mental health and ask your health care professional what medications are safe to take while breastfeeding.

What does baby need?

Mom, there are no rigid rules for breastfeeding that first month. The general guidelines for baby's needs are as follows:

- Feed baby every 2–3 hours during the day. If baby is not awake at three hours, then wake up to feed. If baby sleeps a little longer at night that is fine, but wake baby up to feed if baby sleeps over a 4–5 hour span at night.

- If you're having a hard time waking baby for a feeding, try stripping baby down to his/her diaper for the feeding and caressing baby's body, face, neck, or back. Stroking a clean damp wash cloth over baby's face may also help him or her to wake up.

- Always give baby the full meal deal—feeding at both breasts. Failure to feed baby from both breasts often results in baby being hungry sooner and wanting to nurse again within an hour. By avoiding this "snacking" habit and offering baby the full meal deal, mom and baby will have longer and more regulated breaks between breastfeeding sessions.

- Always look at a clock or watch and take note of when baby begins to feed. If baby begins to nurse at 7 a.m., nurse baby again any time after 9 a.m., but no later than 10 a.m. If you're tired and find it hard to keep track of when baby begins to nurse, make note of these beginning feeding sessions on your smartphone, tablet, or good ol' pen and paper.

- Keep track of which breast you left off at when you ended a breastfeeding session. Begin the next breastfeeding session at this breast. Use a comfortable bracelet or scrunchie on your wrist to signal where you will begin the feeding next time. Don't trust your memory due to sleep deprivation.

- Change baby's diaper before every breastfeeding session—this keeps baby comfortable and helps him or her to wake. Make this practice a habit from the time baby is born through weaning. Enforcing this habit now is key in that you will not have to worry about remembering to change the diaper each time before you breastfeed. Diaper changes will just become an automatic prompt before breastfeeding.

- Feel free to keep your newborn baby in your room at night in a bassinet so you do not have to get up and walk far in your sleep-deprived state. Remember to keep babies safe by putting them on their backs to sleep and in their own bassinet or crib.

What does mom need?

The next things to consider are meeting your needs, mom. To make breastfeeding successful, you're going to need confidence and support. Be assured that breastfeeding IS the best thing you can do for your baby. Its nutritional, emotional, and physical benefits are exactly what your baby needs. If you feel like you're all alone in breastfeeding, please join a breastfeeding support group at your local hospital or in your community. Ask questions and listen to experienced breastfeeding moms. Maybe you have a friend or relative that is breastfeeding or has breastfed and is positive about the breastfeeding commitment and the benefits of breastfeeding. This person is an excellent resource for support and questions you may have.

In addition to confidence and support, mom, you're going to need some time to rest. With all the excitement of baby, visitors, feedings, and diaper changes, you're going to be sleep-deprived and exhausted this month. You're going to need to catch short spurts of sleep whenever you can. I highly recommend napping when your baby naps. Try to catch at least one afternoon nap while baby is napping to help you get through the rest of the day. Because prolactin (the milk producing hormone) levels increase when you sleep, sleeping actually helps you make milk. Please remember that this sleep-deprivation is but a short phase in motherhood, and it too shall pass.

In regard to taking care of yourself, mom, drink extra water and consume more calories. It is only logical that since you're giving fluids to your baby, you will need to replenish these fluids. Especially drink water before every breastfeeding session. Find a water bottle or large cup, fill it with fresh water daily, and put it at your nursing station or at your kitchen counter for a welcome invitation to hydrate. In addition to good hydration, producing milk for baby requires extra calories, so increase your calorie intake with healthy meals and snacks.

To help support your neck and arm muscles while breastfeeding, use your nursing pillow. Although baby is tiny and doesn't weigh much, straining your arms and neck to support baby during multiple breastfeeding sessions every day is taxing. Let the nursing pillow support the baby for you, and keep it by your breastfeeding station so it's ready to help when needed.

Mom, be willing to accept any help people want to give you. If family, neighbors, or friends want to bring you meals, clean your house, do your laundry, run your carpool or anything else—let them! Your body is healing from childbirth and fatigued from newborn motherhood, so let them provide some assistance. Enjoy these generous moments of relief while you can, as the extra help will end soon enough.

What support can dad or the family provide?

Dads often feel like they can't help out much with breastfeeding. True, dad, you cannot produce your own milk, but you can still help support mom in other ways in her commitment to providing the best nutrition for your child.

One way dad can help mom is to do the nightly diaper changes and bring baby to mom for the next feeding. Another way to help is to bring mom drinking water when you hear the baby cry during the night which usually signals that it's time for baby to eat again. Mom's body is healing from childbirth and trying to keep up with milk production. Drinking water is essential for a lactating mom. Another way dad can help is to hold, rock, and soothe an upset baby...especially if baby does not have a wet or dirty diaper and has eaten within the last two hours. New dads may have little confidence in caring for a baby. The best way to alleviate these worries and fears is to help out with baby every day. After all, practice makes perfect!

From meal prep and clean up to errand running and laundry duty, dad can direct and train other family members in how they can be of extra assistance for the good of the family. If seeing things to be done isn't Dad's forte, a honey-do list may be helpful to provide direction.

*"Do not think that love in order to be genuine
has to be extraordinary.
What we need is to love without getting tired."*

- Mother Teresa

The First Month: How Often and How Much?

While I'm not an "expert" in breastfeeding, I do have years of experience breastfeeding in harmony with my own babies' biorhythms. By breastfeeding infants off and on over a period of sixteen years, I began to notice and later expected certain feeding and sleeping patterns. With our second child, I started to notice regular and predictable breastfeeding patterns and sleep biorhythms. I continued these general feeding and sleeping routines with our third and fourth children. With our fifth child, I started to document these feeding and sleeping patterns and routines. When our sixth child arrived, I started documenting pretty much everything. This data helped me realize our babies shared quite similar eating and sleeping biorhythms. It also proved to be a great resource I could reference with our seventh and eighth children— especially when I couldn't remember our other babies' eating and sleeping pattern history.

As newborns, my children nursed approximately 10–15 minutes per breast at both breasts in one feeding session. I found that my babies spit up less and were not overstuffed with milk when I kept their average feeding session per breast at 10–15 minutes. A new feeding session would begin during the day every 2 hours. Night time feeding sessions (which usually began around 10 p.m. when I was good and ready to get some sleep) would span about every 3 hours or more.

At this point, I wasn't concerned about regular naps for baby. If baby was sleepy after a breastfeeding session, I would lay baby down for a nap. I did make a semiconscious effort to lay baby down to sleep after the night feedings of 10 p.m., 1 a.m., and 4 p.m. breastfeedings (see the feeding patterns below) since these were the spans I was trying to get the longest stretches of sleep for myself.

During the first month, your baby will nurse frequently. The number of daily breastfeedings averages around 8 to 12 feedings per 24-hour period. On average, baby is getting 1–2 oz. of milk per breast during a feeding session. This amount may be more or less based on milk production and baby's demand.

Here is what our 6th child's feeding patterns looked like during the first month:

> 6 a.m.; 8 a.m.; 10 a.m.; 12 p.m.; 2 p.m.; 4 p.m.;
> 6 p.m.; 8 p.m.; 10 p.m.; 1 a.m.; 4 a.m. (repeat)

This averaged 10 to 11 breastfeeding sessions per 24 hour day which fell within the recommended guidelines.

Here are some goals for the first month:

- Take each day one day at a time

- Eat, shower, rest, and grab a nap when baby is sleeping

- Begin to establish a feeding and sleeping routine

- Burp baby after feeding at each breast if possible

- Try to stimulate baby with awake time before bed (e.g., songs, talking, or infant massage). I like to target about 30 minutes before baby and I would like to go to bed.

- Let baby sleep longer spans at night if they so desire. This will allow baby to adjust his/her biorhythms and to stretch those night time feeding and sleeping sessions longer.

- If baby is sleepy or sleeping after nursing, lay baby down for a nap or bedtime.

- Do not fret too much about a regular daytime nap routine. Work on getting the nighttime sleeping and feeding patterns down first. We'll focus on daytime naps later.

- Pump a bit of breast milk only if you're engorged and uncomfortable. Your body is producing milk now and sometimes in overabundance. Give your body time to regulate its milk supply for baby. You may store this breast milk in the refrigerator or freezer for future use. Please read and educate yourself on the safe storage of breast milk.

Is my baby really getting enough nourishment to survive?

You may have concerns about baby getting "enough" milk by breastfeeding. It is true that breastfeeding babies are hungry more often. This is because breast milk is more easily digested and moves through the digestive system faster, resulting in breastfed babies eating more often than bottle-fed babies.

Studies have shown that breastfed babies weigh less at one year than formula-fed babies. This weight gap closes by age two. Experts believe that this may be because breastfed babies stop feeding when they are satisfied, unlike formula-fed babies who may be coaxed to finish a bottle and may end up getting more than they need.

A baby growing steadily on a curve over time is the best measure of health.[10] Weighing the baby regularly can show that your baby is getting enough. Nurse visits, support from a doctor, or weigh-ins with a lactation consultant can help moms build confidence that baby is healthy, growing, and thriving.

Key Objectives and Transitions in Months 0–1:

For Mom:
- Marvel at your beautiful new baby
- Take it one day at a time
- Eat, sleep, drink extra water, consume extra calories, and take prenatal vitamins

For Baby:
- 8 to 12 feedings per day
- Breastfeeding every 2 hours during the day
- Breastfeeding about every 3 hours during the night

Transitions:
- Breastfeedings started around 11 times per day at birth and by the end of the month transitioned to about 10 times per day as baby slept longer spans at night
- Try to spread out breastfeeding to 3 hours or more at night to give mom longer spans of rest. To help with this, lay baby down to sleep after nighttime breastfeedings.
- Wake baby during the day if not awake to eat every 2 hours

When, oh, when will my shower come?

Your sweet little angel exudes the fragrance of fresh succulent lavender baby wash. As you breathe, press your nose into baby's soft skin and hair and take in that clean heavenly scent. Maybe you wish that same clean and fresh scent could be had by you.

Unfortunately, after all your new baby help has gone home and your spouse has returned to work, you've been consumed with feedings, catching rest when able, and just trying to keep your head above water on the home front.

Maybe you haven't quite figured out how and when you will be able to shower while keeping tabs on baby. The answer? The baby seat. Whether it's a bouncer, a car seat for younger babies, a Bumbo, a jumper, or an exersaucer for older babies—the baby seat is a must! Put the baby seat right outside your shower door or curtain to keep baby in view while you get cleaned up.

Guide for the Second Month

Congratulations on making it through the first month of breastfeeding! As I tell new breastfeeding moms, "If you can make it through that first month, things begin to get a lot easier." Remember in the past when you began some type of new physical workout routine? (Goodness no, I'm not suggesting you start one now!) Maybe it was riding your bike, running, doing push-ups or sit-ups, or exercising to a workout DVD. Although your muscles ached for days or weeks and it was tough to keep up and catch your breath, you persevered. You did not give up, but pushed through the difficulties and the routine became easier with time.

So it is with breastfeeding. You've made it past the most difficult month with all of its trials. You have persevered, and I'm proud of you! Try to focus on not overdoing it, mom. Just focus on taking good care of yourself so you can best take care of your baby. Adequate sleep for mom is important for mom's health. Hopefully those nighttime feeding and sleeping sessions have stretched out to every three hours at this point so you're getting a bit more rest. If not, don't despair, it will come soon!

Although you may be exhausted and sleep deprived, please do not forget to:

- Drink plenty of water before nursing
- Change baby's diaper before each feeding
- Use your nursing pillow
- Use a bracelet to remind yourself where you left off nursing
- Give baby the full meal deal (nurse at both breasts)
- Burp baby after feeding at each breast if possible
- Keep track of what time you started a feeding session
- Take care of yourself by resting and eating nutritious foods
- Pump a little milk if you feel uncomfortably engorged. Feel free to store this milk following the safe storage of breast milk guidelines found at: www.llli.org

As far as how much and how often baby nurses, somewhere between 5 to 8 weeks, the amount of feedings decreases as napping and sleeping increases. The time nursing at each breast for baby averages about 10 minutes. During the second month, the average number of feedings in a 24 hour period was 9 for our babies.

Here's an example of what our babies' basic feeding and sleeping patterns looked like during the second month:

Breastfeeding	Napping/Sleeping (Duration)
1 a.m.	After Feeding (~3 hrs)
4 a.m.	After Feeding (~3 hrs)
7 a.m.	
	8:30 a.m. (~1 hr)
9:30 a.m.	
	11 a.m. (~1 hr)
12:30 p.m.	
	1 p.m. (~1½ hrs)
3:30 p.m.	
	4 p.m. (~1 hr)
5:30 p.m.	
7:30 p.m.	After Feeding (~1 hr)
9:30 p.m.	After Feeding (~3 hrs)

At this point, the daytime naps were irregular, but the nighttime sleeping sessions of basically 10 p.m.–1 a.m., 1–4 a.m., and 4–7 a.m. were regular (minus feeding times).

Key Objectives and Transitions in Months 1–2:

For Mom:
- Continue to marvel at your beautiful baby
- Keep taking it one day at a time
- Continue to eat, sleep, drink extra water, consume extra calories, and take prenatal vitamins

For Baby:
- 8 to 12 feedings per day
- Breastfeeding every 2½–3 hours during the day
- Breastfeeding about every 3+ hours at night

Transitions:
- Breastfeedings started around 10 times per day at the beginning of the first month and transitioned to about 8 to 9 times per day by the end of the second month as a result of baby sleeping longer spans during the day and at night
- Continue to spread out breastfeeding to 3 hours or more at night to give mom longer spans of rest
- Wake baby during the day if not awake to eat every 3 hours

Please see the appendix at the end of this book for a quick and easy reference guide to baby's average monthly transitions.

"Be faithful in small things because it is in them that your strength lies."

\- Mother Teresa

Guide for the Third Month

From weeks 8 to 12, I noted a significant change in the number of breastfeedings for our children. At around age 8–9 weeks, baby's daily nursing sessions changed from 9 times per day to 8 times per day.

Here are two examples of feeding and sleeping patterns at 8–9 weeks old:

Teresa's Biorhythms:

Breastfeeding	Napping/Sleeping (Duration)
6 a.m.	After Feeding (~1 hr)
8:30 a.m.	After Feeding (~1 hr)
10:30 p.m.	
	11 a.m. (~1 hr)
12:30 p.m.	After Feeding (~1 hr)
	1 p.m. (~1½ hrs)
2:30 p.m.	
	4 p.m. (~1 hr)
4:30 p.m.	After Feeding (~1 hr)
6:30 p.m.	
	7:30 p.m. (~1 hr)
9:30 p.m.	
	10 p.m. (~8 hrs) *(sleeping through the night)*

<u>Calvin's Biorhythms:</u>

Breastfeeding	**Napping/Sleeping** (Duration)
3 a.m.	After Feeding (~3 hrs)
6 a.m.	After Feeding (~3 hrs)
9 a.m.	After Feeding (~1.5 hrs)
12 p.m.	After Feeding (~1.5hrs)
3 p.m.	
5 p.m.	After Feeding (~1 hr)
7 p.m.	After Feeding (~1.5 hrs)
9:30 p.m.	After Feeding(~5 hours)

Although Teresa and Calvin exhibited different biorhythms, the total number of daily breastfeedings was consistent at 8 times per day. Now don't get hung up on the exact times of feedings and naps. As you can see above, one baby may wake earlier or space out their feedings differently from another baby. As far as average time to breastfeed, some of my babies were fast at breastfeeding and nursed an average of 5 to 10 minutes per breast. Some of our other children took their time and nursed slowly for an average of 15 minutes per breast, while others started slowly and picked up their nursing speed as they aged. Sweet baby Teresa slept through the night at 9 weeks while her brother Calvin did not. All babies are unique!

Biorhythms can be adjusted by using a routine of regular feeding and nap times. The important thing to keep in mind is maintaining the number of feeds in a day (in this case, 8) and concluding with that number of feeds by the time you would like to go to bed, mom. My bedtime goal was 10 p.m. What time is the best for you to get your needed rest and rejuvenation? Find a routine that's best for you and continue to work on aligning your and baby's biorhythms.

Be sure to keep baby up for about a half an hour or so before putting baby "officially" to bed at night. This will help baby unwind, allow for awake bonding time with mom and dad, and get baby good and tired before going to bed. Be creative with this with books, songs, and playing. If your baby is not sleeping through the night, that is totally fine. You're still in the process of discovering your baby's biorhythms. As you can see in the above examples within our family, sometimes it just takes longer to figure out. The goal by the end of the third month is to hopefully to stretch baby's sleeping through the night and drop any early morning feeds before 4 a.m.

Just when I thought I had the routine figured out, my babies decided to sleep more at around 10 to 11 weeks and eliminate another nursing, dropping the number of feedings in a day down to 7. See my babies' routine on the following page.

Example feeding and sleeping patterns at 10–11 week old:

Breastfeeding	Napping/Sleeping (Duration)
6 a.m.	After Feeding (~1.5 hrs)
9 a.m.	After Feeding (~1 hr)
11:30 a.m.	After Feeding(~1.5 hrs)
1:30 p.m.	After Feeding(~1 hr)
4 p.m.	After Feeding(~1 hr)
7 p.m.	After Feeding(~1.5 hrs)
9:30 p.m.	After Feeding (~8 hrs) *(sleeping through the night)*

Key Objectives and Transitions in Months 2–3:

For Mom:
- Continue to marvel at your beautiful baby
- Continue to eat, sleep, drink extra water, consume extra calories, and take prenatal vitamins
- Begin to slowly resume normal activities with the approval of your doctor (examples would be lifting items heavier than your baby, resuming a light post-partum routine, etc.)

For Baby:
- 7 to 9 feedings per day
- Breastfeeding every 2½–3 hours during the day
- Breastfeeding hopefully 0–1 times during the night

Transitions:
- Breastfeedings started around 8 to 9 times per day at the beginning of the second month and by the end of the month transitioned to about 7 times per day as a result of baby sleeping longer spans during the day and at night
- Continue to spread out breastfeeding to 3 hours or more at night to give mom longer spans of rest
- Wake baby during the day if not awake to eat every 3 hours
- Drop any early morning feeds before 4 a.m.
- Hopefully baby will be only getting up once per night for a feeding or will be sleeping through the night by the third month

Toddler Afoot: When Moms Exhaust

All moms have good days and not so good days. I remember many times when I was up several times during the night with a baby that was hungry, teething, or sick. It was difficult enough that I was exhausted, but I was also exhausted about keeping up with a toddler child along with a newborn the whole next day.

How would I ever get any rest? I felt like a zombie! There are no easy solutions to this—mostly trial and error and some caffeine. Maybe you can sneak in a quick nap while baby is napping and you're snuggling with your toddler during a favorite show. If your toddler still naps in the afternoon, try and time baby's nap around the same time so you can lie down and rest for a bit.

So maybe it's leftovers for dinner tonight. That is okay. The dirty laundry will always be there tomorrow. If your spouse is home, ask him if he can keep tabs on the little ones while you take a quick power nap and recuperate a little energy. Remember to take things one day at a time. Tomorrow is a new day!

Guide for the Fourth Month

At age 4 months, it is now time to apply what I call the "**3-6 rule**".

The "**3-6 rule**" is something I found to be consistent with all my babies in the fourth month. Basically, the rule goes like this:

The "3-6 Rule"
Baby nurses <u>every **3** hours during the day</u> and requires <u>**6** breastfeedings per day</u>.

However, if baby is nursing more than 6 times per day at four months—that is totally fine. Six feedings per day at age four months is the minimum. Another thing you have hopefully discovered by the fourth month is that baby is sleeping through the night. Mom, this is the point when you're finally able to get more rest and will feel better physically and mentally. With feeling good, you will be able to get back to and focus on the people you love to spend time with and the things you like to do.

Now that baby is hopefully sleeping through the night, you can begin to focus more on a daytime nap routine. Between the third and fourth month, my babies reached a more regular feeding routine of every 3 hours.

Here is the approximate feeding and sleeping routines of our babies at age 4 months—two routines listed to show the variety:

Biorhythm # 1:

Breastfeeding	Napping/Sleeping (Duration)
7 a.m.	After Feeding (~1.5 hrs)
10 a.m.	After Feeding (~1 hr)
1 p.m.	After Feeding (~1.5 hrs)
4 p.m.	After Feeding (~1.5 hrs)
7 p.m.	After Feeding (~1.5hrs)
10 p.m.	After Feeding (~9 hrs)

Biorhythm # 2:

Breastfeeding	Napping/Sleeping (Duration)
6:30 a.m.	After Feeding (~1.5 hrs)
9:30 a.m.	After Feeding (~1 hr)
12:30 p.m.	After Feeding (~1.5 hrs)
3:30 p.m.	After Feeding (~1 hr)
6:30 p.m.	After Feeding (~1 hr)
9:30 p.m.	After Feeding (~9 hrs)

Key Objectives and Transitions in Months 3–4:

Mom, you're doing great! Continue to do the following:

- Snuggle, kiss, talk to, sing to, read to, tickle, marvel at, and love your beautiful baby
- Eat good and healthy foods, get adequate sleep, drink extra water, consume extra calories, and take prenatal vitamins. Breastfed babies are relying on your good nutrition, mom, so they can healthy.
- Resume normal activities and exercise with the approval of your doctor. Resuming your regular routine, mom, will require strength and stamina. Exercise will improve how you feel and help you build back up your strength for lifting baby and all the baby equipment for outings and errands.

From this point forward the above objectives will be referred to as "Mandatory Mom Care."

For Baby:

- 6 to 7 feedings per day
- Breastfeeding every 3 hours during the day

<u>Transitions:</u>
- Begin applying the "**3-6 rule**"
  —breastfeeding every **<u>3</u>** hours, **<u>6</u>** times per day
- Breastfeedings started around 7 times per day at the beginning of the second month and by the end of the month transitioned to about 6 times per day as a result of baby sleeping longer spans during the day and hopefully through the night
- Continue to spread out breastfeeding to 3 hours or more at night to give mom longer spans of rest
- Wake baby during the day if not awake to eat every 3 hours
- Drop any early morning feeds before 4 a.m.
- Hopefully baby will be sleeping through the night by the fourth month

"Love begins at home, and it is not how much we do . . . but how much love we put in that action."

— Mother Teresa

Guide for the Fifth Month

The breastfeeding routine during the fifth month will remain the same during this month. The sleeping routine began to change more this month with longer and less frequent naps.

Here is an example of our babies' feeding and sleeping routines at age 5 months:

Breastfeeding	Napping/Sleeping (Duration)
6:30 a.m.	After Feeding (~2 hrs)
9:30 a.m.	
12:30 p.m.	After Feeding (~2 hrs)
3:30 p.m.	
	5:30 p.m. (~1 hr)
6:30 p.m.	After Feeding (~1.5 hrs)
9:30 p.m.	After Feeding (~9 hrs)

If baby did not wake up by around 9 p.m., I would wake baby up and play, read books, talk, and sing until the final nursing before bed at 9:30 p.m.

Mom, how are you feeling? Are you remembering to take care of yourself with the "Mandatory Mom Care" steps as described in the previous chapter? If you have forgotten what those steps are, please refer back to the last chapter.

Key Objectives and Transitions in Months 4–5:

For Mom:

- Mandatory Mom Care

For Baby:

- Continue applying the "**3-6 rule**"
- Breastfeeding every 3 hours during the day (wake if it's time)
- Total of 6 feedings per day
- Napping less frequently, but in longer spans: about four times per day, usually after each breastfeeding session
- Sleeps through the night

Optimal Performance Preferred:
Moms Need Apply

"I would exercise, but I don't have the time." You've heard it and most likely you've said it. I certainly have. It's tough work being a mom. Moms need to be strong to hold baby, lift other children, carry diaper bags, and load and unload car seats and strollers. All the daily demands of motherhood can leave you emotionally and physically drained. An exercise routine can help you overcome those draining daily slumps. I know when I don't exercise, I'm more tired, lack stamina, and don't feel strong.

The key is finding a time, place, and routine for exercise that works for you. Maybe it's an exercise class at the gym, walking with a friend or spouse, or a video workout program you can do at home. Whatever it is, find a time and routine that works for you and stick with it!

For me, it's waking up a half hour earlier and doing a simple 20–30 minute cardio/strength training video about three times per week. I cue up my Denise Austin DVD the night before, and clear my floor workout space to make the morning transition easier and more inviting. Sometimes I'll add to the workout routine or mix it up with walks outside with my husband or taking a bike ride.

Personally, I know if I don't do the exercise in the morning before the rest of the household wakes up, it won't happen. The hardest part is always getting started. I encourage you to experiment with what works best for you, and commit to feel better and stronger with exercise!

Guide for the Sixth Month

Congratulations, you have made it through half a year of breastfeeding! The time has flown. Your baby is babbling, rolling over, smiling, laughing, maybe sitting up or pushing up, and possibly even trying to crawl. Wow! So much has changed from that tiny little newborn of six months ago. In addition to breastfeeding, at around six months we introduced baby to rice cereal. Bring on the video recorder! We presented cereal at our regular lunch time (between 11 a.m.–12 p.m.) and dinner time (between 5–6 p.m.) In the beginning of the introduction of solids, we would just mix 2–3 tsp. of rice cereal with enough warm water to make it runny. This consistency made it easier for baby to swallow with it not being too thick or pasty. You may also mix warm breast milk with the rice cereal if desired. To feed baby rice cereal, put baby in a high chair, strap on that bib, and spoon-feed baby with a small spoon.

With the transition to solids, our baby didn't eat much at first and spit most of it back out. With time and patience, however, our baby began to catch on to this whole concept of solids and began to eat more. During the sixth month, the number of breastfeedings per day stayed at 6. The napping routine did transition this month from 4 daily naps to 3 daily naps.

Here is an example of our babies' feeding and sleeping biorhythms at age 6 months:

Breastfeeding/ _Solid Food_	Napping/Sleeping (Duration)
6:30/7 a.m.	
	8:30 a.m. (~1.5 hrs)
9:30 a.m./10 a.m.	
11 a.m. Lunch (rice cereal)	
12:30 p.m./1 p.m.	After Feeding (~2 hrs)
3:30/4 p.m.	
5 p.m. Dinner (rice cereal)	
6:30/7 p.m.	After Feeding (~2 hrs)
9:30/10 p.m.	After Feeding (~9 hrs)

If baby did not wake up by around 9 p.m., I would wake baby up and play, read books, talk, and sing until the final nursing for bed around 9:30–10 p.m.

Key Objectives and Transitions in Months 5–6:

For Mom:

- Mandatory Mom Care

For Baby:

- Continue applying the "**3-6 rule**"
- Breastfeeding every 3 hours during the day (wake if it's time)
- Total of 6 feedings per day
- Napping even less: down from four to three times per day
- Sleeps through the night

Transitions:

- May introduce rice cereal mixed with breast milk or warm water

"Love begins by taking care of the closest ones—the ones at home."

\- Mother Teresa

Guide for the Seventh Month

At around seven months, we began baby foods. At the advice of our family doctor, we first introduced baby to the yellow vegetables (squash, sweet potatoes, and carrots), and then the green vegetables (peas and green beans). We introduced vegetables one at a time and didn't switch to any new vegetables until after a few days of observing no allergic reactions. Starting with veggies first encourages babies to eat their veggies and grow accustomed to their flavor first, rather than starting with sweeter fruits and baby rejecting their veggies later.

We served veggies as a meal during our regular lunch and dinner times. One can serve just straight veggies or mix them with some rice cereal. We mixed the veggies with some rice cereal so baby was still getting good vitamins from the rice cereal. At first, baby didn't eat much baby food or fancy its taste. In time however, baby caught on and enjoyed the baby food. What began as baby eating a few teaspoons to a few tablespoons per meal went on to eating ½ jar baby food veggies or more mixed with rice or oat cereal for two meals per day (lunch and dinner).

For the most part, baby's eating and sleeping patterns remained the same as the sixth month. The number of breastfeeding sessions per day stayed at 6. Most of baby's nutrition is coming from mom's milk, so don't feel like you have to overstuff baby with baby food.

Here is our babies' feeding and sleeping biorhythm at age 7 months:

Breastfeeding/ _Solid Food_	Napping/Sleeping (Duration)
6:30/7 a.m.	
	8:30 a.m. (~1.5 hrs)
9:30/10 a.m.	
11 a.m. Lunch _(rice cereal / baby food veggies)_	
12:30/1 p.m.	After Feeding (~2 hrs)
3:30/4 p.m.	
5 p.m. Dinner _(rice cereal / baby food veggies)_	
6:30/7 p.m.	After Feeding (~2 hrs)
9:30/10 p.m.	After Feeding (~9 hrs)

Key Objectives and Transitions in Months 6–7:

For Mom:

- Mandatory Mom Care

For Baby:

- Continue applying the "**3-6 rule**"
- Breastfeeding every 3 hours during the day (wake if it's time)
- Total of 6 feedings per day
- Napping three times per day (about 1½–2 hours per nap)
- Sleeps through the night

Transitions:

- Begin to add baby food vegetables (may mix with rice cereal) for lunch and dinner
- Introduce a new vegetable only after baby has shown no allergic reaction for at least 2–3 days of eating the same one
- As baby becomes more aware and distracted during breastfeeding, mom needs to avoid movement and provide a quiet environment—free of external stimuli

The family meal—more than just eating

Now that baby is eating solids, it is a good time to establish routine meals. Routine meals help establish social interaction within the family, a good time to unwind for all family members, and an avenue for encouraging appropriate table behavior.

Yes, eating "real food" for baby equals more work for mom and dad and more training for baby. There'll be those adorable sticky hands, faces, and messy hair to wipe—not to mention the countless cups, plates, bowls, forks, spoons, and food to clean up that baby hurls to the floor. The good habits we establish now at the family meal will hopefully continue to improve with time. These good habits take many years of practice. Hopefully by the time our little ones leave the nest, they will have it figured out.

We've enjoyed these particular moments of the family meal throughout the years:

- When baby makes funny faces indicating if a new food is liked or disliked
- When family members take turns helping feed baby
- When, after much repetition and modeling, baby finally learns to sign "more" and wait patiently for more food instead of screaming and fussing
- When the dinner table is bustling with noise, goofiness, and excitement as the children share, unwind, and talk about their day
- When good table manners are exhibited by all
- When the family finds their silence for prayer

Guide for the Eighth Month

During the eighth month, four changes in our babies' feeding and sleeping biorhythms were noted. The first was the cessation of the "late" 9–10 p.m. feed. Therefore the "3-6 rule" transitions to baby breastfeeding about every 3 to 4 hours during the day for 5 times per day.* The second was that the number of naps reduced from three to two naps per day. The third was that baby was definitely hungry for a whole jar baby food and would consume it in entirety for both lunch and dinner. Finally, bedtime began earlier at 7 p.m. with baby sleeping through the night until 7 a.m. the following morning.

---

* At 8–10 months, some of our babies still wanted and needed that 6th feeding of the day at 10 p.m. This helped them sleep through the night without waking up in the wee hours of the morning hungry and wanting to nurse. This is totally fine. Remember to tune in to your baby's own *biorhythmic* needs and be flexible. If your baby is not ready to go down to five daily feedings, continue six feedings per day. If you're not sure if baby is ready to go down to five feedings, you may try doing so. If baby wakes up hungry in the wee hours of the morning, continue to feed baby six times per day.

Some of our babies added eating breakfast baby food during this time. Others did not due to being full from the morning breastfeeding in which I had a surplus of milk production from overnight. After several vegetables have been introduced and well-established in the "like" category, you may introduce fruits. I introduced baby food fruits (bananas, apples, pears, etc.) by mixing them into baby's rice cereal for breakfast with a little warm breast milk or warm water. Apply the same introductory rules of waiting 2 to 3 days before adding a new fruit or baby grain cereal to baby's diet to detect any allergies. Baby usually eats anywhere from a half jar to a full jar of baby food at a meal.

As a general rule, orange or yellow veggies were fed during lunch and green veggies were served for dinner. You may also mixed some baby rice/oat/grain cereal into the vegetables for added nutrients. A drink of water may also compliment baby's meal by means of a baby bottle or sippy cup. You may also give your baby breakfast baby food (fruit mixed with oat/rice cereal) for breakfast if baby is still hungry after the 7 a.m. morning nursing session.

If your baby is sitting up by the eighth month, you may also add Cheerios, puffs, or crackers as a tasty snack or supplement while they are eating in the high chair. Breaking these apart at first is helpful as your baby is learning about a whole new texture and the concept of chewing solid food. These foods are good introductory crunchy solids that may be served during family meal times after baby has eaten baby food in the high chair. They help babies to practice their hand–eye coordination, learn about new food textures, and gain experience feeding themselves.

Here is an example of our babies' feeding and sleeping biorhythms at age 8 months:

Breastfeeding/ Solid Food	Napping/Sleeping (Duration)
7 a.m.	
8 a.m. Breakfast (rice cereal / baby food fruit / finger foods)	
	8:30 a.m. (~1.5 hrs)
10 a.m.	
11 a.m. Lunch (rice cereal / baby yellow veggies / finger foods)	
1 p.m.	After Feeding (~2 hrs)
4 p.m.	
5 p.m. Dinner (rice cereal / baby green veggies / finger foods)	
7 p.m.	After Feeding (~12 hrs) [(~2 hrs)]
[10 p.m.] (if baby needs a nightcap to sleep through the night)	[After Feeding (~9 hrs)]

Key Objectives and Transitions in Months 7–8:

For Mom:

- Mandatory Mom Care

For Baby:

- Breastfeeding about every 3–4 hours during the day
- Total of 5 to 6 feedings per day
- Napping two (or three) times per day
- Sleeps through the night

Transitions:

- The "**3-6 rule**" changes to 5 feedings per day (maybe)
- Introduce new foods only after baby has shown no allergic reaction for at least 2–3 days of eating the same one
- Breakfast baby food with baby rice cereal or another grain baby cereal may also be added
- May begin to add baby food fruits
- Baby should be eating more baby food now: half to full jar per meal
- Cheerios may be introduced, if baby is able to sit up unaided
- May serve water in a bottle or sippy cup at mealtime
- When baby is too sleepy to wake up from the 7 p.m. nap to breastfeed, it's time to make 7 p.m. the new bedtime, or baby may still want and need that 10 p.m. feeding

"We can do no great things, only small things with great love."

\- Mother Teresa

Guide for the Ninth Month

The feeding and sleeping pattern remained pretty much the same from the eighth to ninth month. The only changes of note are adding meat as a baby food choice if desired and adding a fruit as a "dessert" after baby ate their normal portion (whole baby food jar) of vegetables for lunch or dinner if he or she still remains hungry. Of course, if baby is hungry after the morning nursing session, you may add baby food breakfast fruit mixed with rice/grain cereal. If desired, add a drink to baby's meal by serving water in a bottle or sippy cup.

Mom, don't forget to continue to take care of your health and nutrition needs while caring for your baby. Continue to drink adequate of water before each breastfeeding session and continue to take prenatal vitamins to supply your baby with nutritious breast milk. Eat regular, well-balanced meals. Help relieve stress and maintain strength and agility to keep up with the demands of motherhood by exercising at least three times per week for 20 minutes.

Enjoy those times during the day when you can sit down, put your feet up and snuggle with your baby. During this special time, try not to be moving, talking, or texting. Mealtimes should be relaxing and precious bonding times for you and your baby. However, today's societal, work, and social pressures often are not conducive to a relaxed environment for nursing baby. It is up to us moms to take a step back, excuse ourselves from what is "expected" and do what is "best" for our children. If baby will not nurse due to distractions from other sources or people in the room, excuse yourself to a quiet place with a comfortable chair and nursing pillow to set the proper atmosphere.

Here are the feeding and sleeping biorhythms of our babies at age 9 months:

Breastfeeding/ _Solid Food_	Napping/Sleeping (Duration)
7 a.m.	
8 a.m. Breakfast (rice cereal / baby food fruit / finger foods)	
	8:30 a.m. (~1.5 hrs)
10 a.m.	
11 a.m. Lunch (rice cereal / baby yellow veggies / finger foods / baby food meats)	
1 p.m.	After Feeding (~2 hrs)
4 p.m.	
5 p.m. Dinner (rice cereal / baby green veggies / finger foods / baby food meats)	
7 p.m.	After Feeding (~12 hrs) [(~2 hrs)]
[10 p.m.] (if baby needs a nightcap to sleep through the night)	[After Feeding (~9 hrs)]

Key Objectives and Transitions in Months 8–9:

<u>For Mom:</u>
- Mandatory Mom Care

<u>For Baby:</u>
- Breastfeeding about every 3–4 hours during the day
- Total of 5 to 6 feedings per day
- Napping two (or three) times per day
- Sleeps through the night

<u>Transitions:</u>
- The "**3-6 rule**" changes to 5 feedings per day (maybe)
- Baby should be eating more baby food (about a whole jar) per meal
- New foods to consider, if baby is ready:
  - Baby food meats
  - Finger foods (e.g., puffs, crackers, etc.)
- Introduce new foods only after baby has shown no allergic reaction for at least 2–3 days of eating the same one
- When baby is too sleepy to wake up from the 7 p.m. nap to breastfeed, it's time to make 7 p.m. the new bedtime, or baby may still want and need that 10 p.m. feeding

> *"Give a man a fish and you feed him for a day;*
> *teach a man to fish and you feed him*
> *for a lifetime."*

Loads of looming laundry. Daunting deposits of dirty dishes. A plethora of piling paperwork. Bedraggled bathrooms. Foul floors. As moms, we've all seen them. What mom isn't overwhelmed with work? From the workplace to work in the home, the to-do list never ends!

When our children are little, we parents pretty much have to do everything. However, sometime around the age of three, a beautiful thing happens. Phrases like, "I can do it myself" and "I want to help" emerge from that sweet little voice. This is an invitation to foster and promote life skills—don't squelch it! You may be tempted to ignore these signs of independence and contributive spirit. Understandable—you can do things much faster on your own. However, if kids are never given the chance to help, how will they ever learn to be independent, accountable, and responsible?

Start out with small tasks your child can do to exhibit their independence and help around the house: folding towels, tidying up toys, getting themselves dressed, and setting the table are all good starters. Continue to increase responsibilities as abilities grow and mature. Go ahead, take the time to look down at your little one and start teaching them how to fish! Guide them along the way and improve their "fishing" with practice and better techniques. Who knows, they might even catch some new fish along the way!

Guide for the Tenth Month

The tenth month signifies the beginning of table foods other than the Cheerios, crackers, and puffs that baby has already sampled. This month, small amounts of table food can be added during all regular meal times in the high chair. At breakfast, we added smashed up bananas mixed into the rice cereal. After serving baby food vegetables for lunch or dinner, we offered small cut up pieces of the family dinner to baby.

Pretty much any safe table food that is not too hard or too chewy can be introduced at meal times during the tenth month. The nap and breastfeeding routine remained the same as it did last month. During this month, baby began to transition from drinking water from a baby bottle during meals to using a sippy cup with water. The tenth month also signified the transition for our babies that were still nursing six times per day to reduce their breastfeedings to five times per day. Baby's bedtime and last nursing of the day became more flexible at night—usually between 7–8 p.m.

Here are the feeding and sleeping biorhythms of our babies at age 10 months:

Breastfeeding/ Solid Food	Napping/Sleeping (Duration)
7 a.m.	
8 a.m. Breakfast (rice cereal / baby food fruit / may begin some table foods)	
	8:30 a.m. (~1.5 hrs)
10 a.m.	
11 a.m. Lunch (rice cereal / baby yellow veggies / may begin some table foods)	
1 p.m.	After Feeding (~2 hrs)
4 p.m.	
5 p.m. Dinner (rice cereal / baby green veggies / may begin some table foods)	
7 p.m.	After Feeding (~12 hrs) [(~2 hrs)]
[10 p.m.] (if baby needs a nightcap to sleep through the night)	[After Feeding (~9 hrs)]

Key Objectives and Transitions in Months 9–10:

For Mom:
- Mandatory Mom Care

For Baby:
- Breastfeeding about every 3–4 hours during the day
- Total of 5 to 6 feedings per day
- Napping two (or three) times per day
- Sleeps through the night

Transitions:
- The "**3-6 rule**" changes to 5 feedings per day (maybe)
- Baby should be eating more baby food (about a whole jar) per meal
- New foods to consider, if baby is ready:
  - Baby food meats
  - Finger foods (e.g., puffs, crackers, etc.)
- Introduce new foods only after baby has shown no allergic reaction for at least 2–3 days of eating the same one
- When baby is too sleepy to wake up from the 7 p.m. nap to breastfeed, it's time to make 7 p.m. the new bedtime, or baby may still want and need that 10 p.m. feeding
- Baby can transition from a bottle of water to a sippy cup of water by the tenth month

"To love, it is necessary to give."

- Mother Teresa

Guide for the Eleventh Month

The breastfeeding and sleeping routine remained the same for baby in the eleventh month as it did during the tenth month. Usually by the eleventh month, baby was satisfied with 5 breastfeedings per day. Baby's added desire for more table food and less baby food is duly noted this month. I continued with baby food fruits and veggies during mealtimes if baby was still receptive. If not, then other table food fruits and veggies were offered to take their place.

At the eleventh month, baby can eat whatever table foods are being served to the family—just cut them in little pieces. If you have a mouth-stuffer, just ration out small portions/pieces while your baby experiments and learns about new textures and flavors. Continue to offer baby a sippy cup with water during meals.

Here are the feeding and sleeping biorhythms of our babies at age 11 months:

Breastfeeding/ _Solid Food_	Napping/Sleeping (Duration)
7 a.m.	
8 a.m. Breakfast _(rice cereal /_ _baby food fruit /_ _table foods)_	
	8:30 a.m. (~1.5 hrs)
10 a.m.	
11 a.m. Lunch _(rice cereal /_ _baby yellow veggies /_ _table foods)_	
1 p.m.	After Feeding (~2 hrs)
4 p.m.	
5 p.m. Dinner _(rice cereal /_ _baby green veggies /_ _table foods)_	
7/8 p.m.	After Feeding (~11–12 hrs)

Key Objectives and Transitions in Months 10–11:

For Mom:
- Mandatory Mom Care

For Baby:
- Breastfeeding about every 3–4 hours during the day
- Total of 5 feedings per day
- Napping two times per day
- Sleeps through the night
- Drinking from a sippy cup of water at mealtimes
- Loves to eat with the family at mealtimes and experiment with new table foods

Transitions:
- Baby may take a shorter morning nap
- Introduce new table foods only after baby has shown no allergic reaction for at least 2–3 days of eating the same one
- A decrease in or cessation of the consumption of baby food occurs

Less is More

There will always be those forces that try and pull us moms away from what is most important. Every day is a constant struggle to stay focused on what matters—our family. If I had to sum up in one phrase what moms need to remember about keeping our priorities clear amid the busyness and distractions of life, it would be: *Less is more.*

Simplifying our family life is the key. How do we as moms do this? Identify and eliminate the "time suckers" and "abundance flooders" in family life. "Time suckers" are those things that keep your family apart both often and for long periods of time.

Three examples of "time suckers" are:
1. Adult's over-commitment to too many activities
2. Child's over-commitment to too many activities
3. Too much technology use

Now don't get me wrong: commitment to something is very good. The problem is when we *over* commit to *too many* things outside the home. This results in stress and the family not being together. Over-commitment is a time sucker that can be eliminated by not being afraid to say "no" or set limits.

Too much technology is another prevalent "time sucker." It's critical that moms and dads establish rules and time limits for technology use for themselves as well as their kids so that family members aren't glowing in front of a screen too long. Building relationships with people face to face is more important than idly wasting time on a screen.

"Abundance flooders" are those tangible things in life that you are drowning in overabundance. There are those occasions that I do not spend time with my loved ones because I am overwhelmed with too much stuff. Clothing that won't fit in drawers and closets, toys that are falling out of the already brimming toy box, and consistent clutter on floors and counters are all obstacles that interfere with a family being comfortable and having an inviting place to work and play.

Avoid these "abundance flooders"—donate unused items to those in need on a regular basis (AMVETS visits my home regularly). In a culture of "more is better," I encourage you to stand firm on the importance of family and drying out your life from these "flooders."

Guide for the Twelfth Month

The one year mark of breastfeeding is a milestone of many measures. You should be proud of providing the best possible nutrition for your baby's first year of life! It wasn't easy and many sacrifices had to be made. You and your baby are happier and healthier because of breastfeeding. Your baby knows he or she is loved and nurtured and can trust you for all physical and emotional needs. Continue to carry on the good work of breastfeeding!

By the end of the twelfth month, baby will most likely be on a complete diet of breast milk and table foods. Overall, baby's nursing and sleeping routine remains consistent with the eighth, ninth, tenth, and eleventh month with a slight reduction in time of the morning nap this month.

Here are the feeding and sleeping biorhythms of our babies at age 12 months:

Breastfeeding/ _Solid Food_	Napping/Sleeping (Duration)
7 a.m.	
8 a.m. Breakfast _(table foods)_	
	9 a.m. (~1 hr)
10 a.m.	
11 a.m. Lunch _(table foods)_	
1 p.m.	After Feeding (~2 hrs)
4 p.m.	
5 p.m. Dinner _(table foods)_	
7/8 p.m.	After Feeding (~11–12 hrs)

Key Objectives and Transitions in Months 11–12:

For Mom:

- Mandatory Mom Care

For Baby:

- Breastfeeding about every 3–4 hours during the day
- Total of 5 feedings per day
- Napping two times per day
- Sleeps through the night
- Drinking from a sippy cup of water at mealtimes
- Loves to eat with the family at mealtimes and experiment with new table foods

Transitions:

- Baby may take a shorter morning nap
- Introduce new table foods only after baby has shown no allergic reaction for at least 2–3 days of eating the same one
- A decrease in or cessation of consuming baby food occurs

Weaning: A Guide for the 13th Month

Now that you've breastfed through baby's twelfth month, I wanted to provide a quick overview of the weaning process and what feedings were eliminated and when. The weaning guide of *Baby Biorhythms and Breastfeeding* is exactly that—a guide. It's a general summary of the average weaning patterns of our children. Weaning is a natural process based on baby's cues. I noticed a reduction in my milk supply during certain normal breastfeeding times of the day, especially once baby started eating table foods regularly. It was during these times that baby breastfed for a very short amount of time (around a minute), was only nursing at one breast for a short amount of time, or just didn't want to breastfeed.

For me, I noted this reduction in milk supply with the mid-morning and mid-afternoon breastfeedings first. The reduction later continued with the mid-day breastfeeding before afternoon naptime. The morning breastfeeding was the second to the last feeding to be eliminated due to baby's disinterest and milk supply reduction. The bedtime breastfeeding was the final breastfeeding to be eliminated due to baby's disinterest and milk supply reduction.

Pay attention to your body and to your baby's breastfeeding demands when deciding how and when to wean. Don't try to wean all at once. Maintain a consistent weaning routine, and note which feedings baby is ready to wean from versus which feedings baby desires to keep.

After one year, baby may drink whole milk with meals or snacks. The paragraphs and charts below provide a quick overview of baby's breastfeeding and weaning biorhythms. Some of our children breastfed longer and others weaned sooner. I averaged their feeding biorhythms below in months 13 to 18. Please do not feel rushed to wean if you and baby are enjoying your breastfeeding time together. Always take things at you and your baby's own pace when weaning.

At around month 13, the 4 p.m. breastfeeding was the first one to be eliminated. Baby continued to be breastfed at the feeding times of 7 a.m., 10 a.m., 1 p.m., and 7 p.m. Normal breakfast, lunch, and dinner times continued with table foods and either whole milk or water to drink. A morning naptime of around 9–10 a.m. and an afternoon naptime of 1–3 p.m. remained consistent. A snack after baby's afternoon nap was added in place of the 4 p.m. breastfeeding. Baby slept through the night from 7 p.m.–7 a.m.

Here are the feeding and sleeping biorhythms of our babies at age 13 months:

Breastfeeding/ _Solid Food_	Napping/Sleeping (Duration)
7 a.m.	
8 a.m. Breakfast	
	9 a.m. (~1 hr)
10 a.m.	
11 a.m. Lunch	
1 p.m.	After Feeding (~2 hrs)
~~4 p.m.~~	
3/4 p.m. Snack	
5 p.m. Dinner	
7/8 p.m.	After Feeding (~11–12 hrs)

Key Objectives and Transitions in Months 12–13:

For Mom:

- Mandatory Mom Care

For Baby:

- Total of **4 feedings** per day
- Napping two times per day
- Sleeps through the night
- Drinking from a sippy cup of water at mealtimes
- Loves to eat with the family at mealtimes and experiment with new table foods

Transitions:

- Introduce new table foods only after baby has shown no allergic reaction for at least 2–3 days of eating the same one
- Add a snack time for baby around 3–4 p.m. to take the place of the 4 p.m. breastfeeding
- Baby may drink whole milk with meals or snacks (Talk to your doctor about what whole milk would be best/right for your baby to meet his/her health needs.)
- Baby can drink from a sippy cup or transition to a straw cup

Weaning: A Guide for the 14th Month

At around month 14, the 10 a.m. breastfeeding was the second one to be eliminated. Baby continued to be breastfed at the feeding times of 7 a.m., 1 p.m., and 7 p.m. Normal breakfast, lunch, and dinner times continued with table food and either whole milk or water to drink. A snack time after the morning nap with finger foods/and whole milk was also added around 10 a.m. The morning naptime of 9–10 a.m. and an afternoon naptime of 1–3 p.m. remained consistent. Baby slept through the night from about 7/8 p.m.–7 a.m.

Here are the feeding and sleeping biorhythm patterns of our babies at age 14 months:

Breastfeeding/ Solid Food	Napping/Sleeping (Duration)
7 a.m.	
8 a.m. Breakfast	
	9 a.m. (~1 hr)
~~10 a.m.~~	
10 a.m. Snack	
11 a.m./12 p.m. Lunch	
1 p.m.	After Feeding (~2 hrs)
3/4 p.m. Snack	
5 p.m. Dinner	
7/8 p.m.	After Feeding (~11–12 hrs)

Key Objectives and Transitions in Months 13–14:

For Mom:

- Mandatory Mom Care

For Baby:

- Total of **3 feedings** per day
- Napping two times per day
- Sleeps through the night
- Drinking from a sippy cup of water at mealtimes
- Loves to eat with the family at mealtimes and experiment with new table foods

Transitions:

- Introduce new table foods only after baby has shown no allergic reaction for at least 2–3 days of eating the same one
- Add a snack time for baby around 10 a.m. to take the place of the 10 a.m. breastfeeding
- Baby can drink from a sippy cup or transition to a straw cup

Weaning: A Guide for the 15th Month

At month 15, the 1 p.m. breastfeeding was the third one to be eliminated. Baby continued to be breastfed at the feeding times of 7 a.m. and 7 p.m. Normal breakfast, lunch, and dinner times continued with table food and either whole milk or water to drink. The 15th month is when baby's morning nap was eliminated.

Baby's naptime moved forward slightly in time from about 12 p.m.–2:30 or 3 p.m. due to baby's earlier tiredness from no morning nap. Baby slept through the night from 7 p.m.–7 a.m.

Here are the feeding and sleeping biorhythms of our babies at age 15 months:

Breastfeeding/ _Solid Food_	Napping/Sleeping (Duration)
7 a.m.	
8 a.m. Breakfast	
	~~9 a.m. (~1 hr)~~
10 a.m. Snack	
11 a.m./12 p.m. Lunch	After Lunch (~2–3 hrs)
~~1 p.m.~~	~~After Feeding (~2 hrs)~~
3/4 p.m. Snack	
5 p.m. Dinner	
7/8 p.m.	After Feeding (~11–12 hrs)

Key Objectives and Transitions in Months 14–15:

For Mom:

- Mandatory Mom Care

For Baby:

- Total of **2 feedings** per day
- Napping **one time** per day
- Sleeps through the night
- Drinking from a sippy or straw cup of water at mealtimes
- Loves to eat with the family at mealtimes and experiment with new table foods

Transitions:

- Introduce new table foods only after baby has shown no allergic reaction for at least 2–3 days of eating the same one
- Eliminate baby's morning nap when baby is restless and alert during this time and no longer sleeps
- Put baby down to nap earlier in the afternoon
- Baby will be tired earlier in the afternoon and hopefully nap longer due to the morning nap being eliminated

Weaning: A Guide for the 16th Month

At month 16, the 7 a.m. breastfeeding was the fourth one to be eliminated. Baby continued to be breastfed between 7–8 p.m. at night (or right before bedtime). Normal breakfast, lunch, and dinner, and 2 snack times continued with table food and either whole milk or water to drink. Baby had one naptime per day after lunch beginning between 12–1 p.m. until about 2:30 or 3 p.m. Baby slept through the night from 7/8 p.m.–7/8 a.m.

Here is the feeding and sleeping routine for the 16th month:

Breastfeeding/ Solid Food	Napping/Sleeping (Duration)
~~7 a.m.~~	
8 a.m. Breakfast	
10 a.m. Snack	
11 a.m./12 p.m. Lunch	After Lunch (~2–3 hrs)
3/4 p.m. Snack	
5 p.m. Dinner	
7/8 p.m.	After Feeding (~11–13 hrs)

Key Objectives and Transitions in Months 15–16:

For Mom:
- Mandatory Mom Care

For Baby:
- Total of **one feeding** per day
- Napping one time per day
- Sleeps through the night
- Drinking from a sippy or straw cup of water at mealtimes
- Loves to eat with the family at mealtimes and experiment with new table foods

Transitions:
- Eliminate the 7 a.m. breastfeeding
- Introduce new table foods only after baby has shown no allergic reaction for at least 2–3 days of eating the same one
- Eliminate baby's morning nap when baby is restless and alert during this time and no longer sleeps
- Put baby down to nap earlier in the afternoon
- Baby will be tired earlier in the afternoon and hopefully nap longer due to the morning nap being eliminated

Weaning: A Guide for the 17th Month and Beyond

Sometime around 17 months of age or more, the 7 p.m. breastfeeding was the last one to be eliminated. Weaning is hard to do—especially when you and baby look forward and enjoy that one-on-one snuggle time together. When you and baby are ready to wean, give baby a sippy cup with water and create a bedtime ritual of rocking or reading a story while baby sips from a sippy cup to continue that one-on-one snuggle time with mom and/or dad. One afternoon naptime continued from this age through age 2½ to 3 for our children. Bedtime continued to be between 7/8 p.m.–7 a.m.

You may be asking yourself, when should I wean? There are no set rules. My personal guidelines for weaning are:

1. Once the baby is over 12 months old and isn't interested or struggles during nursing sessions

2. When the baby only nurses for a minute or two, or only for a short time at one breast and isn't getting much breast milk

3. Once maternal instinct senses "it's the right time"

Key Objectives and Transitions in Months 16–17+:

For Mom:

- Mom, continue to take care of yourself by eating right, getting adequate rest, and exercising.

For Baby:

- Baby is eventually weaned
- Napping one time per day
- Sleeps through the night
- Drinking from a sippy or straw cup of water at mealtimes
- Loves to eat with the family at mealtimes and experiment with new table foods

Transitions:

- Eliminate the 7 p.m. breastfeeding
- Introduce new table foods only after baby has shown no allergic reaction for at least 2–3 days of eating the same one
- Eliminate baby's morning nap when baby is restless and alert during this time and no longer sleeps
- Put baby down to nap earlier in the afternoon
- Baby will be tired earlier in the afternoon and hopefully nap longer due to the morning nap being eliminated

Congratulations, Graduate!

You did it—well done! Congratulations on your perseverance with breastfeeding to provide your baby with the best health benefits possible!

You questioned. You researched. You studied.
You prepared. You practiced. You practiced some more.
You observed. You transitioned. You navigated.
You implemented. You evaluated. You adapted.
You endured. You improved. You prioritized.
You breathed. You balanced. You modeled.
You believed. You bonded. You loved.

You left a legacy!

You've proven by hard work and example that breastfeeding baby within a biorhythmic routine can and does work. Not only have you touched the life of your baby as well as your own, but you've inspired the lives of those around you.

Your witness will encourage other moms to nurture their own conviction to breastfeed. Lactation consultant and mother, Amber Hinds, puts this sentiment best in her article in the Huffington Post when she was challenged for breastfeeding at a public pool:[7]

"We still have far to go regarding the normalization of breastfeeding in this country. How important it is for us as mothers to be confident in our choices and to be able to stand up for ourselves and our children. I could have moved to the locker room, but I didn't because I knew that I wasn't doing anything of which I should be ashamed or that should be hidden. I was caring for my baby in the best way that I know how and I was setting an example of motherhood not just for my daughters, but for every girl and young woman there."

Now, I challenge you to be a beacon of hope and a pillar of fortitude. Shine your light on other moms as they navigate through these unclear and unchartered waters!

Q&A, Tips, and Resources

Here are some questions, answers, tips, and resources about baby, biorhythms, and breastfeeding.

Q: My child is not a good breastfeeder. According to baby's doctor, my child is not gaining enough weight. Baby's doctor recommends formula supplementation and possibly the cessation of breastfeeding.

Do you have any recommendations before giving up breastfeeding?

Since you have already spoken with your doctor, the next step is to meet with a lactation consultant or a La Leche League leader right away about proper latch on techniques and ways to increase your milk supply. Contact your local hospital to get in touch with a certified lactation consultant. Increasing one's milk supply often involves breastfeeding more often and for longer spans. Supplementation will definitely decrease your milk supply since baby will be nursing less.

Q: What are some causes of low milk supply?

Common causes of low milk supply may be improper latch-on and infrequent nursing caused from formula supplementation. Two excellent articles to ready are "How Can I Increase My Milk Supply?" and "Hidden Hindrances to a Healthy Milk Supply." Both articles are by Becky Flora who is an International Board Certified Lactation Consultant.

Q: I need to take X medication(s). My doctor recommends that I stop breastfeeding so the medication is not in the breast milk.

What should I do?

One resource is the book titled "Medications and Mother's Milk" by clinical pharmacologist, Dr. Thomas W. Hale. In his book, Dr. Hale notes that "with most medications, the amount transferred into human milk is generally low."

Dr. Hale further notes that "there are almost always other medications that could be substituted for that are safe for both mother and infant." So why are moms being told to stop breastfeeding due to use of medication? Dr. Hale states that "The pharmaceutical manufacturer's resistance to using medications in breastfeeding mothers is almost always based on legal reasons not clinical ones." "Because the PDR (Physician's Desk Reference) lists only the pharmaceutical's package insert, the standard recommendation is to not take the medication while breastfeeding. The PDR is the poorest source for obtaining accurate breastfeeding information." [6]

A second resource to research medications is the Drugs and Lactation Database (**LactMed**) from the National Institute of Health's Library of Medicine, available online at:

http://toxnet.nlm.nih.gov

This database is updated monthly, and has information on the levels found in breast milk and infant blood, as well as possible adverse effects on nursing infants. Where appropriate, it also includes suggested alternatives that may allow you to continue to breastfeed while needing a prescription medication.

Use these resources to research your medications and discuss any findings or alternatives with your doctor to make a more informed decision on the best health choices for you and your baby.

Q: *Will I be able to breastfeed and still work outside the home or leave for extended hours or an overnight?*

That answer depends on how committed you are to breastfeeding. If you're able to excuse yourself during the workday to a private area to pump breast milk and have a place to store it, then most certainly! As long as your baby will take a bottle from your spouse or caregiver, and you're able to pump and store, you can continue to breastfeed.

Did you know that there is <u>federal law</u> called the "Break Time for Nursing Mother's Law" that requires employers to provide break time and a place for hourly paid workers to express breast milk?

Communicate with your employer in advance about your intentions to pump breast milk upon returning to work and what accommodations can be made—a break to pump breast milk, a private area to do so, and a safe place to store it. If your employer is not accommodating, do your homework on your federal and state rights and present these facts in a kind way.

Q: What if my baby isn't following the example eating and sleeping biorhythms?

Every baby is unique. The example eating and sleeping biorhythms are just that—examples. You will need to discover your baby's eating and sleeping biorhythms and adjust/align them with your own. The main thing to consider is making sure baby is receiving a **consistent** and **necessary number of feedings per day** and not be hung up on the exact times of those feedings.

Q: Should I add vitamin drops to my baby's diet? Will my baby be iron deficient without vitamin drops?

Doctors vary on the answer on the answer to these questions in regard to the health of the baby. It is true that babies get most of the needed vitamins and minerals from breast milk if their mothers are taking a pregnancy/lactation vitamin daily and eating a healthy, well-balanced diet.

Mom can ensure that baby is getting adequate iron by taking care of herself, taking her prenatal/lactation vitamin, adding an iron supplement if recommended by her doctor, and feeding baby fortified iron rice cereal at or after 6 months of age.

Q: What do I do if baby is sick or having a growth spurt? Should I break from the routine?

The routine is only a guide and definitely not rigid in its following. Many a baby has woken up in the middle of the night with a fever that was soothed with some pain medication and breastfeeding. The last thing you want your baby to become is dehydrated, especially when sick. Mom, your amazing body knows what baby needs and will adjust and compensate. It will also readjust after that time of need has passed. The same goes for when baby is having a growth spurt and wakes up for an occasional nighttime feeding that is not part of the normal routine. It is totally fine to breastfeed your baby when this occurs.

Q: Should I breastfeed baby if I am sick?

According to pediatrician Alanna Levine, under most circumstances, it is safe to breastfeed if you're sick. With a standard cold, flu, or stomach bug, or even a fever, it is usually fine to breastfeed. Baby has been exposed to the illness before you even began to show symptoms. Since your body is ramping up its immunity to fight the illness, those antibodies will help protect your baby when you breastfeed.[11]

Q: What do I do if baby is distracted and will not breastfeed?

Find a quiet place for you and baby that is free from exterior noise, people, and distractions. If you're in an environment in which that objective is difficult to achieve, try and cover baby with a blanket for a tent-like effect that will hopefully shield from outside stimuli.

Q: Can I tweak the breastfeeding routine?

Most certainly. Here are a few of examples:

Scenario # 1:

Let's say you have a wedding to go to, but it's time to feed the baby now. You're short on time before the wedding starts and don't want to have to feed the baby in the middle of the ceremony. So, give the baby feed a "half meal deal" (from one breast) to tie him or her over during the ceremony, and give him or her the "full meal deal" (from both breasts) after the ceremony when you can find a quiet place and have more time for nursing.

Scenario # 2:

You and your spouse would like to go on a date some evening and would like to leave before that 7 p.m. nursing and bedtime. You don't want to worry about pumping and having a sitter feed the baby. It is fine to push your feeding times up during the morning and afternoon to accommodate. So instead of feeding at 7 a.m., 10 a.m., 1 p.m., 4 p.m. and 7 p.m., you can start baby's feedings earlier to look something like this: 6:30 a.m., 9:30 a.m., 12:30 p.m., 3 p.m., 6–6:30 p.m.

<u>Scenario #3:</u>

Baby is now eating baby food at regular meal times in conjunction with the regular breastfeeding routine. You're on a trip and baby is fast asleep in the car. Instead of waking baby, you decide to drive an extra hour. Doing this, however, pushes the baby food lunchtime or dinnertime close to the next nursing session. Should you first breastfeed or give baby food to baby upon stopping?

The answer I give to this is something I call "the flip." Once baby is well established in a normal breastfeeding and baby food routine, it is totally fine to "flip" these feedings if they are falling awfully close together. In this circumstance, I recommend breastfeeding baby first, followed by serving baby food. This way, baby is getting what is really important first—breast milk.

Q: Should I give my baby juice?

According to the American Academy of Pediatrics, babies younger than 6 months should not be given juice. Too much juice can cause diarrhea, diaper rash, promote tooth decay, and contribute to obesity. It is better to give babies that are eating table foods whole fruits that provide better nutrition. If you do offer your baby over 6 months of age juice, make sure it is 100% juice, no more than 4 ounces per day, given only with a snack or meal, and served only in a cup and not in a bottle. In addition to following the above guidelines by the AAP, I also heavily dilute juice given to baby with water.

Q: Everyone keeps telling me to start feeding baby foods earlier and that my baby looks hungry.

How do you respond to pressures from society to not breastfeed in public or exclusively breastfeeding until 6 months of age?

I'll borrow a phrase from Scott Adams that my husband likes to use: "Get the apathy cream!"

If I need to breastfeed in public, I will. If others are uncomfortable with my breastfeeding in public, I just ignore them. Better to make others uncomfortable than deny my baby sustenance.

As far as exclusive breastfeeding until 6 months, whenever society starts chiming in that I must be "starving" my baby by withholding baby food, I kindly reply, "the doctor says my baby is growing just fine. Did you know the American Academy of Pediatrics now recommends that exclusive breastfeeding is best for infants until at least 6 months of age?" I then kindly smile.

Q: My baby has abruptly stopped or significantly reduced normal biorhythmic breastfeeding and struggles when I try to nurse.

Why is baby doing this? Is it time to wean? How can I get my baby back to regular breastfeeding?

Your baby may be having a nursing strike. The reasons for a nursing strike are often unclear. A few common causes are teething, illness, and distractions while nursing. Unless baby is over the AAP recommended age of 12 months for breastfeeding, I encourage you to stick out the strike and keep on trying! A nursing strike may last a few days to a few weeks or more.

Express or pump breast milk to avoid engorgement and try offering baby breast milk in a cup. If your baby is at least 12 months of age and is still uninterested in breastfeeding after a few weeks of expressing or pumping breast milk, then it may be time to wean. When it is time to wean, do not quit breastfeeding or stop pumping breast milk all at once. Follow the weaning guide as suggested in this book—even if you need to pump to reduce your milk supply and eliminate breastfeeding sessions without baby's input in the matter.

I wish I had known what a nursing strike was eleven years ago. At that time, my 11-month-old son abruptly quit nursing and refused the breast entirely for three days. I thought he was just ready to wean and ended up doing so.

Three excellent articles to read to learn more about nursing strikes and get tips to help both you and baby during this difficult time are:

1. "My Baby Is Suddenly Refusing to Nurse. Does That Mean It's Time to Wean?" http://www.llli.org/faq/strike.html

2. "Is Baby Weaning or Is It a Nursing Strike?" http://www.llli.org/nb/nbnovdec92p173.html

3. "Surviving a Nursing (Breastfeeding) Strike" by Becky Flora http://www.motherandchildhealth.com/Breastfeeding/Becky/strike.html

Q: What should I do if baby bites me while breastfeeding?

Teething is the most common reason for baby to bite. Baby may be in pain and is testing out those new/emerging teeth. As hard as it sounds, try not to yell or startle baby. If baby does not let go, insert your index finger into the corner of baby's mouth and between the back jaw gums to loosen baby's clenched jaw and remove your nipple.

Q: My baby does not always want the "full meal deal" (breastfeeding from both breasts) at a nursing session. What should I do?

For younger babies, falling asleep at the tap is common. Use the methods described earlier in **The First Month: Beginning Breastfeeding** to help baby wake up and complete the full meal deal. This not only keeps baby satisfied, but keeps mom comfortable and avoids engorgement.

For older babies (over 6 months), avoid exterior distractions and stimuli while nursing. If baby refuses to nurse at the second breast during a breastfeeding session, wait 15 minutes or so and then offer the second breast. Another thing I have found helpful is to space breastfeedings farther away from mealtimes—keeping them about 1–2 hours apart. If baby has filled up on baby or table foods, he or she may not be hungry for breast milk until later.

For babies around or over 12 months of age, reducing the amount of desired breast milk or only wanting to nurse at one breast at a nursing session may be a sign that baby is slowly beginning to wean. To avoid breast engorgement or the "favoring" of one breast, do switch which breast is offered at every nursing session and always offer the second breast—even if it is rejected. When it is time to wean, do not quit all at once. Follow the weaning guide as suggested in this book.

Q: *My baby is over 12 months old and doesn't want to nurse as much or as often, and I'm getting engorged. Should I be pumping milk?*

Yes, it is fine to pump milk to relieve the engorgement. If baby is weaning and refusing to nurse at certain feeding sessions of the day, pump milk during the time of the dropped or refused feeding. Pumping enough milk to relieve your discomfort should be adequate. Breast milk supply is regulated based on a natural "supply and demand" balance: the greater the demand for milk (i.e., the more you pump or express), the more milk the body will supply. Likewise, the lesser the demand for milk (i.e., the less you pump or express), the less milk the body will supply. You will want your milk supply to diminish naturally during those cut feedings with time. To achieve this, do not pump too much milk or your body will think it needs to make more. At the same time, do not pump too little milk or get to the point that you're painfully engorged.

Q: *What is mastitis and what should I do if I get it?*

Mastitis is when a plugged milk duct or a sore breast becomes infected. Mom will feel weak, achy, tired, and may have fever and chills. It is important for Mom to breastfeed baby frequently to alleviate swelling and breast pain and to help open up the blocked area of the breast. Plenty of rest for mom and applying heat to the sore breast(s) (e.g., taking a warm shower in which to massage the breast) will help unplug the blocked duct. If after 24 hours of frequent nursing, rest, and heat, mom is still feverish and uncomfortable, contact your healthcare professional. An antibiotic may be needed. If an antibiotic is prescribed, continue frequent breastfeeding, rest, and heat treatments during recovery.

For more information, visit www.llli.org.

Q: *When should we move baby to his or her own room?*

As a general couple's rule, we moved baby to his or her own room sometime between the ages of 10 to 12 weeks. For us, it was easier and more convenient to keep baby in our room in the bassinet those first couple of sleep-deprived and nursing-plenty weeks. By week 12, baby was sleeping longer spans and nursing less often at night.

We also slept better by not hearing all those cute little baby noises that kept us sleeping very lightly—well maybe at least one of us. By maintaining our own sleeping biorhythms, we felt we could provide more attentive care for our precious new baby than in exhausted mental and physical states.

Q: What can I do to make an outing with baby less stressful and preparation less time-consuming?

First, keep a well-stocked diaper bag with an extra change of clothes for baby in every vehicle you drive. This will take the guess work out of "what to pack" for baby's outing and save time.

Second, if you're going to be out for a couple of hours or longer, have everything ready and plan to leave *immediately after* baby's breastfeeding session. This will give you more time for travel and errand running before that next breastfeeding session.

Q: Where can I get support and more information about breastfeeding benefits, tips, techniques and troubleshooting?

La Leche League International: `www.llli.org`

La Leche League USA: `www.lllusa.org`

American Academy of Pediatrics: `www.aap.org`

Contact your local hospital or lactation consultant to inquire about a breastfeeding support group in your area.

Appendix: Biorhythm Transitions for Baby

This appendix provides a summary of the biorhythm transitions that baby will experience over time from birth until he or she is finished breastfeeding and eating table food. Next is a month-by-month outline of dietary fluids, sleeping patterns, and new food transitions. However, please use these only as a guideline, not as a hard milestone or rigid timeline. Each of our own children progressed differently through these transitions, but all generally followed the same overall flow. As discussed earlier in this book, the recommendation trends for when to introduce certain food types or fluids may change and individual baby dietary preferences vary—make your own informed decisions for what will be best for you and your own baby.

0–6 Months: Drink, Sleep, and Repeat

The 0–6 month old baby's needs consist of drink, sleep, and repeat. Begin at birth by breastfeeding about every 2–3 hours on demand and around the clock. Work toward helping baby adjust to day and night biorhythms by consistently breastfeeding baby at more evenly spaced 2–3 hour intervals during the day and allowing baby to sleep for increasingly longer spans at night as baby desires (3–5 hours).

You will note a transition by the decrease in the number of daily breastfeedings when your baby wants to sleep more and for longer spans at night. By about 3 months of age, baby can breastfeed every 3 hours, for 6 or more times during the day and is hopefully sleeping through the night (8 hours or more).

Daytime napping is sporadic at first since the focus is on helping baby adapt and establish a nighttime sleeping biorhythm. Once baby is sleeping well at night (and so is mom), mom can focus on noting the daytime patterns of baby's sleepiness and begin to lay baby down for regular daytime naps at around 4–5 months of age with an average of 3–4 daily naptimes per day.

6–12 Months: Drink, Sleep, Eat, and Repeat

The 6–12 month old baby's needs consist of drink, sleep, eat, and repeat. At six months, baby continues to breastfeed about every 3 hours, 6 times per day. Starting at around 6 months of age, baby can begin rice cereal, followed by other grain cereals in addition to breastfeeding. Between 7–10 months of age, baby can begin eating baby foods in addition to breastfeeding. At around 10 months of age or older, baby can begin eating table foods in addition to breastfeeding.

During months 6–12, you will most likely note other transitions such as: baby sleeping longer at night, baby being awake more during the day, and baby consuming more baby foods or table foods at regular mealtimes. This may result in baby's breastfeedings spanning longer from every 3–4 hours during the day and reducing in number to 5 times per day.* Baby's short daytime naps will most likely combine to longer and less frequent naps resulting in about 2 per day—morning and afternoon.

---

* Although this pattern held true for most of our children, we had one that would not sleep for more than an 8 hour span at night. To synchronize biorhythms, mom gave him a nightcap at 10 p.m. so she could get her 8 hours of rest to do her job best the next day

13 Months and Beyond: Drink, Sleep, Eat, Repeat...Wean

The 13 month old and older baby's needs consist of drink, sleep, eat, repeat, and eventually to wean. Continue to breastfeed baby every
3–4 hours during the day and feed baby table foods at regular mealtimes. You may notice that if baby takes a morning nap, that baby isn't tired for an afternoon nap. You may further notice that with no afternoon nap, baby is a fussy mess. If this is the case, help baby transition out of the morning nap and push the prominent nap to the afternoon.

Baby may also be showing signs of weaning. Weaning is a gradual process and each baby will wean at his or her own pace. Do not stop breastfeeding all at once. Baby will let you know which nursing sessions to eliminate first based on disinterest or lack of demand—breastfeeding less than usual or showing little or no desire to nurse at all. Wait a week or more before dropping the next breastfeeding time. When you notice that baby is only nursing for a minute or two at one or both breasts during certain regular breastfeeding times, or just isn't interested in nursing at certain regular breastfeeding times, it may be time to eliminate that feeding.

I noticed a reduction in milk supply due to a lack of baby's demand first at the mid-afternoon breastfeeding session followed by the mid-morning breastfeeding session. These were the first two breastfeeding sessions to be eliminated for me. The early afternoon breastfeeding before naptime was the third to be eliminated due to baby's disinterest or lack of demand. The first breastfeeding of the morning was the fourth breastfeeding session to be eliminated followed by the last breastfeeding before bedtime.

Dietary Fluids:

- **0–1 month:** breast milk every 2 hours during the day and spread out breastfeeding at night to 3 or more hours; breastfeeding about 8–12 times per day

- **1–2 months:** breast milk every 2–3 hours during the day and spread out breastfeeding at night to 3 or more hours; breastfeeding about 8–12 times per day

- **2–3 months:** breast milk every 2½–3 hours during the day; breastfeeding about 7–9 times per day

- **3–4 months:** breast milk every 3 hours during the day; breastfeeding about 6–7 times per day

- **4–5 months:** breast milk every 3 hours during the day; breastfeeding about 6 times per day

- **5–6 months:** breast milk every 3 hours during the day; breastfeeding about 6 times per day

- **6–7 months:** breast milk every 3 hours during the day; breastfeeding about 6 times per day; water in bottle or sippy cup to help wash down rice cereal

- **7–8 months:** breast milk every 3–4 hours during the day; breastfeeding about 5 or 6 times per day; water in bottle or sippy cup to help wash down rice cereal and baby foods

- **8–9 months:** breast milk every 3–4 hours during the day; breastfeeding about 5 or 6 times per day; water in a sippy cup to help wash down baby foods and snacks

- **9–10 months:** breast milk every 3–4 hours during the day; breastfeeding about 5 or 6 times per day; water in a sippy cup to help wash down baby foods and snacks

- **10–11 months:** breast milk every 3–4 hours during the day; breastfeeding about 5 or 6 times per day; water in a sippy cup to help wash down table foods

- **11–12 months:** breast milk every 3–4 hours during the day; breastfeeding about 5 times per day; water in a sippy cup to help wash down table foods

- **12–13 months:** breast milk every 3–4 hours during the day; breastfeeding about 5 times per day; water or whole milk in a sippy cup to help wash down table foods

- **13–14 months:** breast milk about 4 times per day; water or whole milk in a sippy cup at snack and meal times

- **14–15 months:** breast milk about 3 times per day; water or whole milk in a sippy or straw cup at snack and meal times

- **15–16 months:** breast milk about 2 times per day; water or whole milk in a sippy or straw cup at snack and meal times

- **16–17 months:** breast milk about 1 time per day; water or whole milk in a sippy or straw cup at snack and meal times

- **18+ months:** baby is weaned; water or whole milk in a sippy or straw cup at snack and meal times

Sleeping Patterns:

- **0–1 month:** after breastfeeding sessions

- **1–2 months:** after daily breastfeeding sessions for about an hour and about every 3 hours after nighttime breastfeeding sessions for about 3 hours

- **2–3 months:** after daily breastfeeding sessions for about an hour and about every 5–8 hours after the nighttime breastfeeding session(s)

- **3–4 months:** after daily breastfeeding sessions for about 1–1½ hours and about 8 or more hours after the nighttime breastfeeding session

- **4–5 months:** about 4 naps per day for about 1–2 hours each and sleeping through the night

- **5–6 months:** about 3 naps per day for about 1½–2 hours each and sleeping through the night

- **6–7 months:** about 3 naps per day for about 1½–2 hours each and sleeping through the night

- **7–8 months:** about 2 to 3 naps per day for about 1½–3 hours each and sleeping through the night

- **8–9 months:** about 2 to 3 naps per day for about 1½–3 hours each and sleeping through the night

- **9–10 months:** about 2 to 3 naps per day for about 1½–3 hours each and sleeping through the night

- **10–11 months:** about 2 naps per day of 1½–2 hours each and sleeping through the night

- **11–12 months:** 2 naps per day of 1–2 hours each and sleeping through the night

- **12–13 months:** 2 naps per day of 1–2 hours each and sleeping through the night

- **13–14 months:** 1 to 2 naps per day of 1–2 hours each and sleeping through the night

- **14–15 months:** 1 nap per day of about 2–3 hours and sleeping through the night

- **15–16 months:** 1 nap per day of about 2–3 hours and sleeping through the night

- **16–17 months:** 1 nap per day of about 2–3 hours and sleeping through the night

- **18+ months:** baby is weaned, and hopefully afternoon napping continues for quite awhile

New Foods:

When introducing new foods to baby, present them one at a time for 3 days before switching to another new food to help identify any possible food allergies. Avoid trying baby food mixtures of multiple ingredients until baby has had a chance to try them separately with no allergic reactions.

- **0–6 months:** breast milk, breast milk, and more breast milk

- **6–7 months:** Rice/grain cereal mixed with warm water or breast milk at mealtimes. Slowly begin baby food vegetables at mealtimes.

- **7–8 months:** Rice/grain cereal may be mixed with baby food vegetables or fruits at mealtimes. Begin small pieces of Cheerios.

- **8–9 months:** Rice/grain cereal may be mixed with baby food vegetables or fruits at mealtimes. Continue with introduction of small finger foods (e.g., Cheerios, crackers, puffs, etc.)

- **9–10 months:** Rice/grain cereal may be mixed with baby food vegetables/fruits/meats at mealtimes. Continue with introduction of small finger foods (Cheerios, crackers, puffs, etc.) By the tenth month, small portions of the family table foods may be cut up and offered to baby at mealtimes.

- **10–11 months:** Rice/grain cereal may be mixed with baby food vegetables/fruits/meats at mealtimes. Table foods in small pieces and finger foods.

- **11+ months:** Table foods in small pieces

Bibliography

1. "Breastfeeding Overview." *WebMD.com*. Web MD, LLC. 2014. Web. 24 June 2014.

2. Brown, N., Gellar, C., & Kazbour, C. "Breastfeeding Experience Survey Outcomes." *pamf.org*. Palo Alto Medical Foundation. 15 Oct. 2013. Web. 24 June 2014.

3. Dermer, Alicia. "A Well-Kept Secret Breastfeeding's Benefits to Mothers." *New Beginnings*. Vol.18 No. 4, July-August 2001. Web. 4 July 2014.

4. Eidelman, A. I., & Schanler, R. J. "Breastfeeding and the Use of Human Milk." *pediatrics.aapublications.org*. American Academy of Pediatrics. 27 Feb. 2012. Web. 24 June 2014. (doi: 10.1542/peds.2011-3552)

5. "Greek/Hebrew Definitions (philoteknos)." *Bibletools.org*. Church of Great God. 2014. Web. 24 June 2014.

6. Hale, Dr. Thomas. *Medications and Mothers' Milk*. Amarillo: Pharmasoft Publishing L.P., 2014. Print.

7. Hinds, Amber. "Why I'm Glad Someone Told Me To Stop Breastfeeding In Public." *HuffingtonPost.com*. TheHuffingtonPost.com, Inc. 17 April 2013. Web. 24 June 2014.

8. Houdmann, S. Michael. "What does the Bible say about Christian mothers?" *GotQuestions.org*. Got Questions Ministries. 2014. Web. 24 June 2014.

9. "How can I tell if my baby is getting enough milk?" *LLI.org*. La Leche League International. 29 Oct. 2006. Web. 24 June 2014.

10. "Is it true that breastfed babies grow more slowly than formula-fed babies?" *Babycenter.com*. Dec. 2013. Web. 25 Sept. 2014.

11. Levine, Alanna. "Is it safe to breastfeed if I'm sick?" *Babycenter.com*. June 2012. Web. 2 Sept. 2014.

12. Lothian, Judith A. "The Birth of a Breastfeeding Baby and Mother." *The Journal of Perinatal Education*. 14(1), 2005. Web. 24 June 2014. (doi: 10.1624/105812405X23667)

13. McCarthy, Dr. Claire. "The top four reasons moms stop breastfeeding-- and what we can do about them." *Boston.com*. Boston Globe Media Partners, LLC. 4 June 2012. Web. 24 June 2014.

14. Moon, Rachel Y. "SIDS and Other Sleep-Related Infant Deaths: Expansion of Recommendations for a Safe Infant Sleeping Environment." *pediatrics.aapublications.org.* American Academy of Pediatrics. 2011. Web. 24 June 2014. (doi: 10.1542/peds.2011-2285)

15. "More Mothers Are Breastfeeding." *cdc.gov.* Centers for Disease Control and Prevention, 07 Feb. 2013. Web. 09 Nov. 2014.

16. "Progress in Increasing Breastfeeding and Reducing Racial/Ethnic Differences—United States, 2000–2008 Births." *MMWR.* 2013;62:77-80. Centers for Disease Control and Prevention. Web. 09 Nov. 2014.

17. Spock, Dr. Benjamin. *Baby and Child Care.* New Revised and Enlarged Edition. New York: Pocket Books. 1968. Print.

18. "What are the benefits of breastfeeding my baby?" *LLLI.org.* La Leche League International. 17 Nov. 2006. Web. 24 June 2014.

19. "Why Breastfeeding is Important." *Womenshealth.gov.* Office on Women's Health, U.S. Department of Health and Human Services. 4 Aug. 2011. Web. 24 June 2014.

Additional References

Adams, Scott. *dilbert.com.* 1 April 2001. Web. 29 Sept. 2014.

Flora, Becky. "Hidden Hindrances to a Healthy Milk Supply." *motherandchildhealth.com.* Web. 29 Sept. 2014.

Flora, Becky. "How Can I Increase my Milk Supply?" *motherandchildhealth.com.* Web. 29 Sept. 2014.

Scolozzi, Fr. Angelo. *Thirsting for God.* Ann Arbor: Servant Publications. 2000. Print.

Online References

www.aap.org

www.ewtn.com

www.goodreads.com

www.llli.org

toxnet.nlm.nih.gov

www.usbreastfeeding.org